W9-ACP-216

Praise for BALANCED NUTRITION:

"A sensibly balanced look at a grossly unbalanced public health campaign mounted by the National Institutes of Health and the American Heart Association, but aided and abetted by the media. It is high time the public learned to recognize the difference between facts and fantasies on the cholesterol issue; this book has the facts, and is an easily read and readily understandable summary of what's known—and even more important—what is *not* known."

Edward H. Ahrens Jr., M.D., The Rockefeller University

"This objective analysis of relations between nutrition and health provides a long overdue counterbalance to the barrage of misleading information on diet and disease to which Americans have been subjected in recent years."

Alfred H. Harper, Ph. D., Former Chairman,
Food and Nutrition Board, National Research Council

"A must. Written by three scientists with superb credentials who are not afraid of going against conventional wisdom."

F.J. Francis, Ph. D., Past President,
Institute of Food Technology

"This well written and authoritative book is exactly the sort of sanity that's needed in current discussions of a very confused subject."

Thomas N. James, M.D., Past President,
American Heart Association

BALANCED NUTRITION

Beyond the Cholesterol Scare

BALANCED NUTRITION

Beyond the Cholesterol Scare

Fredrick J. Stare, M.D.
Founder, Department of Nutrition,
Harvard School of Public Health

Robert E. Olson, M.D.
Professor of Medicine
State University of New York at Stony Brook

Elizabeth M. Whelan, Sc.D.
President,
American Council on Science and Health

BOB ADAMS, INC.
PUBLISHERS

ISBN: 1-55850-997-6 (paperback)
ISBN: 1-55850-920-8 (cloth)

Published by Bob Adams, Inc.
260 Center Street, Holbrook MA 02343.

Printed in the United States of America.

10 9 8 7 6 5 4 3 2 1 Cloth
10 9 8 7 6 5 4 3 2 1 Paper

This publication is designed to provide accurate information with regard to the subject matter covered. It is not, and is not intended to be, a substitute for consultation with a qualified physician. If medical advice or other expert assistance is required, the services of a competent professional in the field should be sought.

ABOUT THE AUTHORS

Fredrick J. Stare is Professor Emeritus and founder of Harvard's Department of Nutrition. He is well known for his numerous books, articles, and papers in the field of nutrition, and for some years wrote the popular column "Food and Your Health," published by the Los Angeles Times Syndicate.

Robert E. Olson is professor of medicine and pharmacological studies at the State University of New York at Stony Brook. He was twice the recipient of Guggenheim Foundation awards, and also received the Joseph B. Goldberger Award in Clinical Nutrition from the American Medical Association. Dr. Olson is past chairman of the Food and Nutrition Board, National Research Council.

Elizabeth M. Whelan is president of the American Council on Science and Health, a national, nonprofit educational group that promotes objective, scientifically validated evaluations of food, chemicals, and health. She is the author of numerous books on nutrition and health.

Acknowledgments

The authors would like to thank Kathy Meister and Brandon Toropov for their help in the preparation of this book.

Dedication

To the responsible professionals in medicine, public health, and the media who are committed to the dissemination of accurate health information.

CONTENTS

Introduction / 19

Section One:
Nutrition in the Spotlight / 29

Chapter One: A Brief History of Eating / 31

A summary of the development of nutrition as a science. What did the ancients think about food—and why? What were the most important scientific breakthroughs? What diseases are diet-based? What myths and superstitions still surround our diet today?

Chapter Two: "Good" Foods, "Bad" Foods / 49

Why we must look at the entire diet, rather than any single part of it: no food is good or bad in and of itself. Do diets that emphasize one food heavily really work? Are hormones used in processing our beef dangerous? Does oat bran "cure" heart disease?

The main difference between health foods and other foods is (surprise!) the price. Do strict vegetarians face any potential health problems? What dangers are associated with health food products? What does "organic" really mean? Can some chemical additives used in standard food products actually protect your health?

Why the current food scares (including the controversy about Alar in apples) say more about journalistic irresponsibility than they do about any real threat to public health. How safe is the American food supply compared to that of other countries? Is the use of saccharin dangerous? How safe is tap water compared to bottled water? What risks are really associated with preparing food?

Cholesterol is essential for all animal life. What purpose does it serve in the human body? Is cholesterol synonymous with heart disease? What about dietary fats?

An objective look at the nation's number one killer. What is coronary heart disease, and what causes it? Are other factors besides cholesterol more important in assessing risk? What are the risk factors we can control? How important are health problems like obesity, high blood pressure, and smoking with regard to heart disease? Are there factors beyond our control that may influence the likelihood of suffering from coronary heart disease? Who is most at risk?

Chapter Seven: Diet and Cholesterol Beyond the Scare / 139

There is no such thing as a "cholesterol cure"—because cholesterol isn't a disease! Cholesterol itself—the fatty substance—is neutral with regard to risk; the key question is how our bodies process it. Half of the population cannot alter serum cholesterol levels through dietary changes of any kind; for those in the controversial "borderline high" group, there is no evidence of decreased coronary heart disease mortality through dietary changes. Why the current serum cholesterol risk categories are designed to alarm, rather than inform. Some of the most prestigious medical organizations in the country are recommending sweeping changes in the American diet—changes that will have no positive effect on the risk of heart disease for most citizens.

Chapter Eight: Why the Cholesterol Hype Is Hazardous / 163

A look at the advantages, from a public health standpoint, of treating those individuals genuinely at risk—rather than attempting to diagnose the entire country simultaneously. Are we exaggerating the risks facing the general public? Why should we make people who are not at risk feel needlessly guilty about eating? Are there more pressing health problems to spend the money on?

Section Three: What Do We Eat? / 177

Chapter Nine: Obesity and Overweight / 179

The many serious health risks associated with obesity: conquering the "malnutrition of the affluent." What's the best way to reach—and maintain—a reasonable weight? What kinds of diets can actually be dangerous? What are the health risks associated with putting children and infants on low-fat diets? How important is exercise? Is it really possible to lose weight from a single "problem area"? Why is it dangerous to lose a great deal of weight in a short period of time?

Chapter Ten: For Women Only / 213

How do the nutritional needs of men and women differ? How can diet affect one's risk of osteoporosis? What are the effects of rigid dieting during pregnancy? What special needs do pregnant or breastfeeding women have? How can pregnant women be sure they're minimizing risks to the fetus? What causes anorexia nervosa and bulimia?

Chapter Eleven: Eating Right in a Complicated World / 225

How can we be certain we're eating a balanced diet? What are the Basic Four Food Groups—and why is it important to eat foods from these groups? What are the essential nutrients? Are vitamin supplements necessary for good health?

Chapter Twelve: Food on the Run / 247

Eating right is easy, even if your lifestyle is a hectic one. How do processed foods differ from fresh ones? How nutritious are convenience foods? Can "microwave cuisine" be a part of a balanced diet? What about people who skip breakfast?

Chapter Thirteen: Day by Day / 261

Enjoyable, balanced, seven-day meal plans for most adults who want to lose pounds or maintain their current weights.

INTRODUCTION

We wrote this book to address the unfounded concerns many people have about the safety and quality of the American food supply.

Today, many of us are alarmed when we even hear the word "cholesterol" in connection with our diets. We are often led (incorrectly) to associate serious risks to human health with the consumption of foods treated with agricultural chemicals such as Alar, a growth regulator used safely by the apple industry since 1967. The wide variety of alleged toxins, carcinogens, and contaminants in many other foods can also give rise to a great deal of anxiety. The concerns even extend to the saccharin we use to sweeten our coffee, and, for that matter, to the coffee itself!

This underlying fear of food is coupled with a general distrust of the very government agencies that exist to protect our food supply—agencies such as the Food and Drug Administration (F.D.A.), the United States Department of Agriculture (U.S.D.A.), and the Environmental Protection Agency (E.P.A.). Thus, when dark rumors or dramatic charges about our food appear, the typical response is a "knee-jerk" assumption that the allegations are based on fact—followed by horror. The net result is often widespread panic, some compelling media exposure for the proponent or proponents of the original (and usually seriously flawed) position, little or no responsible rebuttal of the allegations, and a renewed skepticism of the safety and healthfulness of the food supply.

What little discussion there is of nutritional matters in the mass media, then, often represents generous servings of perspective-free, high-drama, low-information, artificially inflated "fast news." Is it any wonder that food phobias have become so common?

The reality is that our food supply is the best, safest, and most nutritious of any in the world. The government agencies charged with overseeing this high quality are, on the whole, doing an excellent job.

That these facts are not generally known is, in part, the result of the print and broadcast media's willingness to generate publicity for irresponsible charges—assuming, of course, that the charges can hold the interest of an audience. However, physicians and scientists who maintain silence in the face of sensational inaccuracies must also share some of the blame.

In writing this book, we hope to encourage responsible health professionals to favor science over headlines, in-person diagnosis and treatment of diseases like coronary heart disease over ineffective "mass medicine," and responsible health advice over unproven short cuts.

We believe many of the most prestigious medical organizations in the country have made ill-advised and irresponsible decisions on a number of important contemporary health issues. Consider the following.

Item:

In 1988, The American Cancer Society published what was described as "the first-ever cookbook from the national American Cancer Society," with the clear (but unsupportable) implication that eating according to the society's menus would keep one from developing cancer. The book's title, "A Menu for Good Health: The American Cancer Society Cookbook," certainly did nothing to dispel the popular but incorrect notion that certain foods can prevent or cure cancer. A headline in a public service announcement prepared by the Society read, "A defense against cancer can be cooked up in your kitchen." Promotional materials for the cookbook carried an endorsement from the Director of the Division of Prevention and Control, National Cancer Institute, which read in part, "Using this book, people can eat well knowing they are following guidelines that may help them reduce their risk of getting some cancers." We wonder how many people noticed the words "may" and "some" in the above quote. The fact is that the links between diet and cancer are extremely tenuous ones, and the American

Cancer Society's cookbook probably did more to further the cause of food faddism than it did to promote awareness about cancer. What exactly is gained by misleading the public in this way?

Item:

In 1989, the National Academy of Sciences' task force on Diet and Health recommended the most stringent general dietary modifications yet. They advise that all persons, regardless of the presence or absence of risk indicators for coronary heart disease such as serum cholesterol levels, blood pressure, and smoking, should go on restricted diets. Why should groups such as premenopausal women and preteen children, who are virtually immune to coronary heart disease, make such drastic dietary changes?

Item:

By lending its name to the high-visibility "Count Out Cholesterol" campaign, the American Medical Association has taken advantage of the financial support of major food and drug companies. These companies, of course, have a vested interest in selling people their products —whether or not the people reading the backs of the cereal boxes are at risk for coronary heart disease! What public health benefit is attained through this questionable marriage of medicine and commerce?

We have no desire to debunk legitimate, well-informed public health efforts regarding cancer, coronary heart disease, or any other chronic illness. It seems quite clear, however, that the initiatives outlined above simply reinforce the inaccurate stereotypes people have about food: namely, that some foods have miraculous curative powers, while others (such as foods containing cholesterol) are "bad for you" regardless of what the rest of your diet looks like. Such obfuscation is neither good medicine nor good science, and it certainly is not the best use of the limited public health resources available.

The medical and public health professions have no corner on the market for misleading or oversimplified health information. In February 1989, the Natural Resources Defense Council, a group made up primarily of lawyers, not scientists, released a report claiming that trace levels of agricultural chemicals posed what they called an "intolerable" risk of cancer to humans, particularly children. The report focused on Alar, an agricultural chemical found in some apples.

The concentrations in question were considerably below existing government-established safety levels. The media, nevertheless, had a field day, and the consequences were immediate and dramatic. Apple sales plummeted. Panicked consumers threw out wholesome food. Some schools went so far as to ban apple products for a time. Large-scale economic disruption resulted in apple-producing regions. For a while, people actually seemed to worry more about apples as a cause of cancer than about cigarettes!

As will become abundantly clear later in this book, about the only constructive thing the media-fueled fear about apples contributed was higher news ratings and increased newspaper and magazine sales. The reality is that there has never been a case of ill health related to the use of Alar—or any other agricultural chemical—when the chemical in question is used in a regulated, approved manner.

Does our food contain levels of harmful residues of pesticides, hormones, and other toxic or carcinogenic chemicals sufficient to cause illness? In short, is our food supply poisoned? We think not.

Are we doing a good job of educating ourselves and our children about nutrition? We think not. For all the headlines, food scares, and fad diets, the degree to which Americans possess an adequate knowledge of what we eat and what good nutrition means often leaves much to be desired.

This book incorporates the best facts currently available about balanced nutrition. We offer what follows in the hope that readers will be able to achieve better health through better nutrition.

We recognize (as many in the health professions seem to have forgotten) that eating is one of the pleasures of life and that it is unnecessary and unwise to recommend dramatic dietary changes that serve no purpose. Diet changes may be advisable for high-risk individuals in an attempt to reduce their risk factors for certain diseases (specifically coronary heart disease), but such changes are not, in our opinion, warranted for the entire U.S. population.

In conclusion, we quote from "Toward Healthful Diets," published by the National Research Council/ National Academy of Sciences, in 1980. One of us (REO) was the principal author of this publication.

"In a sound program of preventive medicine, appropriate nutritional guidance is an essential part of a comprehensive plan involving immunization, improvement of physical fitness, prevention of accidents, and avoidance of cigarette smoking, alcohol [and other drug] abuse. . . . [With regard to coronary heart disease,] surveillance of risks by health professionals is recommended for all healthy persons. . . . The Board expresses its concern over excessive hopes and fears in many current attitudes toward food and nutrition. Sound nutrition is not a panacea. Good food that provides appropriate proportions of nutrients should not be regarded as a poison, a medicine, or a talisman. It should be eaten and enjoyed."

Fredrick J. Stare, Ph.D., M.D.
Boston, Massachusetts

Robert E. Olson, Ph.D., M.D.
Stony Brook, New York

Elizabeth M. Whelan, M.P.H., Sc.D.
New York, New York

SECTION ONE: NUTRITION IN THE SPOTLIGHT

Chapter One: A Brief History of Eating

A Brief History of Eating

Nutrition in perspective

How have human diets changed over the centuries? What health risks related to food did our forebears face? When and how did the science of nutrition develop? What advances have been made in recent years? The answers to these questions can help us appreciate the many strides made over the centuries in what we know about food, and may also make it easier to understand some of the current myths and misperceptions associated with our diet.

A brief history of eating

What was man's prehistoric diet?

In prehistoric times, food gathering and hunting were major human activities. Our ancestors' diet consisted mostly of animals, fruits, nuts, leaves, roots, and other readily collectible edible items. For some of these early cultures, animal products made up about thirty-five percent of the diet, while plant products made up the remainder. Other cultures ate meat almost exclusively. The diet depended chiefly on the location of the population and the availability of foodstuffs.[1,2,3]

About 10,000 years ago, with the development of agriculture, the human diet changed and expanded. Farming was perhaps the first significant event to change the way people ate. A great deal of trial and error was undoubtedly required for humans to reach this stage.

Why do we attach near-magical properties to some foods, and shun others?

This should really come as no surprise; through the ages, people have learned by observation and experimentation which foods can serve as good sources of nutrition and which are harmful. People have learned to choose food carefully. Perhaps as a protective reflex, humans seem to apply strong taboos to certain foods and to attribute tremendous curative and other health-related properties to others. These attitudes may say more about sociology and anthropology than they do about the food we've eaten over the centuries.

Instincts about "good" and "bad" foods, then, are by no means isolated developments in one or two prehistoric cultures. In actuality, these perceptions are part of the social functioning that has been associated with foods for as long as the human race has existed.

Do myths about our food persist today?

Indeed, for many this quasi-mysticism still exists. Even in our current society, different foods are, at various times, attributed almost magical qualities, while others are shunned, seemingly without reason, as immoral, poisonous, or unhealthy. This will probably always be a feature of human life, regardless of what we now know about the importance of looking at foods in balanced groups, rather than individually, and regardless of the massive amounts of information that exist to disprove the most fanciful theories.

Today, for instance, some attribute "cures" of major diseases to individual foods—such as oat bran, cereals, and vegetarian diets as a "cure" for heart disease and other disorders. Such oversimplistic ideas, usually fueled by minimum research and maximum media exposure, tend to persist no matter how much the scientific community tries to place the issues on a sounder footing. Though oat bran can have a minimal cholesterol-lowering effect in *some* persons, it does nothing to offset important risk factors like smoking or obesity and is not a magical weapon against coronary disorders.

As for "bad" labels currently applied without reason to our food, we usually need look no further than the headlines of the daily newspaper. The recent apple scare, treated at length elsewhere in this book, serves as a modern example of mass hysteria over a completely harmless and nutritious food.

We are perhaps not so far removed from prehistoric man as we might believe.

"Gifts from the gods"

How important was diet to the ancients?

In ancient times, food was considered a gift of the gods. It's easy to see why: people were, broadly speaking, primarily at the whim of the elements as far as their food was concerned. It seems logical enough that communities or tribes would account for the abundance or lack of food in terms they could understand.

If a drought or flood caused a break in the food supply, what other conclusion was a primitive culture to reach than the obvious one—that an angry god was punishing the people for misdeeds?

The calamities associated with nature's disruption of the human food supply can still carry tremendous implications, but humans have learned to anticipate and moderate these events with the aid of science. The attainment of this state of knowledge took many centuries, however, and a general ignorance of the role the environment played in food production—and that of dietary effects on human life—would persist over a vast period of time.

If the dark periods of ignorance were long ones, however, bright light would, over time, be turned on the long-held superstitions about food.

What we eat, what it means

How did knowledge about our food finally advance?

Like many other areas of human knowledge, nutrition has undergone dramatic advances in recent history. What follows is a brief account, from the eighteenth century to the present, of the development of the field of nutrition from myth and fantasy to the science that it is today. The last three centuries have seen more rapid improvements in the overall health and development of the human race than any other period in history. This is due in no small part to the strides humans have made in understanding what we eat and how it affects our health.

In the early 1700s, it was generally believed that each type of food contained a nutrient, a medicine, and a poison. Even when experiments were shown to contradict these beliefs, the evidence wasn't enough, at that time, to change the minds of those who studied food.

How did early nutritionists misread information about the human diet?

Because physicians believed that each food had only one nutrient, the advancement of the study of foods was severely limited. The scientists of the era, it seems, were so devoted to this simple idea that they were content to "wear blinders" and ignore or rationalize away troublesome contradictions—as well as promising new ideas. Any change in this attitude was extremely slow to evolve.

For instance, James Lind, a British naval doctor, discovered in 1747 that scurvy, a deadly disease marked by bleeding gums and spots on the skin, could be cured by adding fresh fruits and vegetables to the diet. This development, however, was not pursued by scientists in any meaningful way for almost 200 years.

The first steps

In Paris in the late 1700s, Antoine Lavoisier's experiments with respiration proved that oxygen is absorbed by the body and carbon dioxide and water are given off, and that this happens in both humans and animals. With this discovery came the realization that the energy needed to carry on bodily functions is a product of the process of combustion, or the "burning" of nutritive elements in food.

How were foods first analyzed?

As the nineteenth century dawned, many of the archaic beliefs of the past persisted. The stage was set, however, for more scientific discovery. This period marked the beginning of chemical analysis of foods—the detailed study of the chemical makeup of foods from both plant and animal sources.

One of the most profound discoveries arising from this work finally addressed the troublesome question of what exactly is *in* foods. Carbohydrates, fats, and proteins, all of which are nutritionally important, were finally recognized as more significant factors than the archaic nutrient-medicine-poison model. It was believed (and later proved conclusively) that carbohydrates and fats fuel the body.

How did we learn about the nutritive values of foods?

The progress continues: chemical analysis

A pioneering German researcher, Justus von Liebig, believed that through chemical analysis he could estimate the nutritive value of different foods. This was disputed as early as 1850. Liebig also concluded that the nutritive value of proteins depends on their nitrogen content. This was to be challenged in the next century; nevertheless, Liebig's work was taken as the basis of much of the future research.

Other important discoveries in the nineteenth century concerned the minerals iron, calcium, and phosphorus. Iron, it was finally learned, is necessary to the formation of blood; calcium and phosphorus were found to play integral roles in bone growth. In addition, scientists were beginning to realize that milk contained essential trace nutrients, but they were, as yet, unidentified.

Although these discoveries and others have stood the test of time, the accepted method of exploration of the nineteenth century, chemical analysis, is no longer the primary weapon at the disposal of scientists. Chemical analysis was supplemented with other types of investigation, notably the biological method of analysis. This approach entails feeding two groups of animals a given diet, both with and without a given supplement—and monitoring (primarily) the results of the different diets on growth.

In this way, research was broadened substantially. Instead of simply studying the elements within a food sample, scientists could now measure the effect different foods had on a growing organism, such as a laboratory rat. The new approach yielded a number of important discoveries.

How many vitamins are there? How were they identified?

In the early part of the twentieth century, scientists learned, for instance, that there are many trace nutrients in foods essential to the prevention of disease. Originally called "accessory growth factors" by F.G. Hopkins at Cambridge University, these food substances were later called vitamins (or "life-giving" chemicals). These discoveries confirmed the finding of James Lind on scurvy and supported the earlier belief that elements found in fresh fruits and vegetables were a necessary part of the diet. A total of thirteen vitamins were identified, a group that now comprises an alphabetical family including vitamin A, the B-complex vitamins, and vitamins C, D, E, and K. Researchers also found that different proteins played different roles in the promotion of growth.

What health advances can be attributed to the growth of knowledge about nutrition?

Many serious health problems common even as late as the early part of the twentieth century were found to occur as the result of poor nutrition. Fortunately, the discovery of vitamins in foods, and the realization that they were necessary for good health, led to the eradication of many diseases.

It is a sign of the remarkable advances in nutrition science that so many of the diet-based diseases that plagued populations in the comparatively recent past are now virtually unknown in developed countries. Following is a partial list of the human diseases for which there are nutritional cures.

What causes the major diet-based diseases?

Anemia (a deficiency of red blood cells and hemoglobin; victims show pallor and are weak) Treatment: iron and vitamin B_{12}, found in meat products, and folic acid, found in spinach and other dark green, leafy vegetables *[Note: iron-deficiency anemia is one of several types of anemia.]*

Goiter (an enlargement of the thyroid gland characterized by severe swelling in the front of the neck) Treatment: iodide, found in iodized salt

Pellagra (a disorder marked by problems in the nervous system, severe skin rash, mental changes, and other symptoms) Treatment: niacin, a B-complex vitamin, found in meats, poultry, fish, enriched and whole-grain cereals, and other foods

Rickets (a disease affecting children that involves failure in bone development) Treatment: vitamin D and calcium, both of which are found in fortified milk

Scurvy (a disorder associated with swollen gums, shortness of breath, and spots on the skin) Treatment: vitamin C (ascorbic acid), found in fruits and vegetables

Xerophthalmia (a disease of the eyes, skin and lungs—still the leading cause of blindness in Asia) Treatment: vitamin A and carotene, found in green and yellow vegetables

Over the centuries, hundreds of thousands of deaths have been attributed to these diseases; yet many individuals today are unaware that they even exist!

Consolidating gains

Once scientists began to discover the cures for these diseases, research identified at least 50 nutrients as necessary for human growth.

There are other ways in which the advancement of nutritional research has helped dramatically to improve health statistics. In the United States at the turn of the century, for example, the infant mortality rate was as high as 10 percent of all live births. That statistic is now down to 1 percent of all live births, and much of the improvement can be attributed to an increased emphasis on good prenatal nutrition.

Life expectancy in the early 1900s in this country was only about 50 years. This has increased to between 73 and 80 years in the United States and other industrialized nations, in part because of improved dietary practices. (Of particular importance in recent years has been the development of the Basic Four Food Groups, guidelines for nutrition education that are discussed in detail on pages 227–230.)

In addition, the quality of our lives has been substantially improved through increased understanding of the foods we consume. One example would be the pasteurization of milk, a process that significantly reduces the danger of spoilage and contamination by dangerous bacteria. Similarly, chlorination and filtration eliminate the disease-causing bacteria in our water supply.

The American food supply of the late twentieth century presents an amazing variety of dietary choices. Furthermore, the foods we consume are more nutritious than those consumed only a few generations ago, because products are often fortified and enriched.

More Americans than ever before are now reaching their full growth and age potentials. In many ways, this is the result of far better nutritional practices than were common through most of human history.

A good time to be alive

As the industrialized nations work to translate their gains into initiatives that can benefit populations of underdeveloped countries, the next chapter in the history of nutrition is being written. The advances made in the study and science of the human diet have substantially changed the lives of every member of the human race. Most of these changes have been for the better—decreased infant mortality, increased life expectancy and quality of life, control and prevention of disease, and the recognition and acceptance of a regimen of nutrients necessary for proper growth.

What are the implications of extending human life to near its "genetic potential"?

Ironically, because people are now living longer, they are living long enough to develop the diseases of middle and old age, including heart disease, stroke and cancer—leading causes of death among older adults. Nutritionists and other scientists now turn their sights to these challenges.

Of course, other advances in public health (notably improvements in sanitation and the development of vaccines to combat infectious diseases) have played important roles in improving life expectancy. For most of us, however, the improved quality of our diet remains one of the most tangible signs of our progress in enhancing the quality of life.

Those of us who are lucky enough to live in this era should realize how profound the relatively recent changes in human nutrition have been. As we've seen, the improvements in diet and public health have been truly remarkable. Especially in the United States, where the quality and variety of the food supply contributes significantly to our high standard of living, the gains have been dramatic when viewed over the last fifty years alone.

We have made major strides with regard to nutrition—though food faddism and quackery remain with us to this day. To some degree or another, however, most of us receive important basic information about what is and is not nutritionally sound in our diets. It is up to each of us to learn more about balanced nutrition, take advantage of this knowledge, and live by it.

Chapter Two: "Good" Foods, "Bad" Foods

Myths and misconceptions

As we have seen, there are a number of widespread myths and fanciful beliefs associated with our food. Many of these attitudes are deeply rooted in human nature and likely to remain long-term features of the way humans look at what they eat.

In this chapter, we'll take a look at some of the implications accompanying common misconceptions about the American diet. There's probably no better place to start than the subject of the ubiquitous "miracle diets."

Do diets that emphasize one food work?

Losing weight... or perspective?

If you're one of the millions of Americans trying to lose excess body weight, you already know that there are some odd weight loss programs to choose from.

Many of the more sensational diets—the type likely to appear on the cover of a tabloid newspaper—focus exclusively on one food. You've probably seen these headlines; they're the ones that trumpet something like "Amazing Radish Weight Loss Program" or "Startling Low-Calorie Tomato Soup Diet." Presumably, the idea is that a diet that emphasizes one or two foods will be easier to understand (and more successful in selling newspapers) on a mass level than one that features more complicated guidelines. Nutritionally, however, such diets dominated by a single food are nonsense.

Beyond panaceas and poisons

These diets, like so many other pieces of media-inspired nutrition advice, perpetuate the "good food/bad food" myth.

It would be a much simpler world if we could say with confidence that cholesterol is "bad for you" and that oat bran is "good for you"—at any level of consumption, in any setting, for anyone. And certainly such simplistic notions are implied regularly in the tabloids and elsewhere. But things are, of course, not that simple.

Are any foods "good" or "bad" on their own?

There is no such thing as a good or a bad food. The term "junk food" is a meaningless one, as it is virtually always used to describe a single dietary item—and not the entire range of foods a person eats.

Carrots, for example, could be considered a bad food. They are usually thought to be a food that contributes to good health, which indeed they are—if consumed as part of a balanced diet. However, if you consume huge amounts of carrots for any extended period, you will develop carotenemia, an unpleasant condition that features, among other things, a transformation in the color of the palms of your hands and the soles of your feet from their normal tone to a bright orange. In this case, carrots have as much claim to the "junk food" label as anything in the snack or cookie aisle of your supermarket.

Similarly, there are few if any parts of a standard, balanced American diet that are, in and of themselves, harmful. Anything can be misused, but conversely any food is good if it is used in a moderate, balanced diet. The dichotomy between "health food" and "junk food," then, is a misleading one. The question is not whether a single food is present in the diet but whether the diet, taken as a whole, conforms to accepted nutritional guidelines. In the case of most of the "miracle diets" found on the pages of supermarket tabloids, there's little doubt that other sources can present better nutritional advice.

Does oat bran prevent heart disease?

Oat bran

While we're discussing the "good food/bad food" myth, it's probably worthwhile to note that the extravagant claims associated with a currently stylish food, oat bran, are overstated.

There is no scientific evidence directly linking oat bran with a decreased risk of coronary heart disease. Oat bran does have some cholesterol-lowering effect, but not much. It is definitely not a substitute for a properly planned, medically prescribed, cholesterol-lowering diet. The irony of this fad is that some of the oat bran cereals actually have higher levels of fat and total calories than competing brands. It's likely that the net health benefit of oat bran products is minimal.

If you are overweight or a smoker, you would do better to lose some weight or quit smoking than to eat a lot of oat bran. Regular blood pressure checks and scrupulous attention to medically prescribed treatment for high blood pressure are also extremely important. We should note, too, that despite the emphasis placed on diet by many books, articles, and television programs these days, ***heredity,*** not diet, plays a predominant role in the likelihood of developing coronary heart disease. (This and other topics related to coronary heart disease will be discussed in detail later in the book.)

Why has oat bran become so popular?

Why has the oat bran fad become so popular? The most obvious answer is that a few million dollars' worth of marketing can make even a fuzzy idea a commonly accepted one. Fundamentally, though, the question is, why do we want to believe such things about our food?

By now, that answer should be apparent. People tend to look to food as either a poison or a panacea. Neither pole really presents the best vantage point.

Many consumers, having been presented with a small amount of information based on very limited research, have apparently decided to look at oat bran as a panacea. Fiber, it seems, is a very "in" dietary substance, and serum cholesterol levels are becoming a concern for many. Combine the two, and you have a new (and successful) marketing wrinkle.

Do high-fiber diets lower the risk of cancer?

Fiber itself certainly seems to fall into the "good food" category these days. One of the most popular claims of the food faddists is that fiber reduces the risk of certain types of cancer.

There is no convincing evidence that high fiber diets, in and of themselves, reduce the risk of cancer. Most societies in which such a link has been claimed are societies where people don't live long enough to develop the type of cancer being studied!

Certainly, fiber is a necessary part of a complete diet. It is important, but definitely not necessary (or advisable) in voluminous amounts. Nevertheless, because the "fiber factor" is a currently trendy subject, its importance is often exaggerated.

Some people believe, for instance, that it is not healthy to eat white bread because there is little fiber in it. If white bread were the only source of food in your diet, that would be a real problem, but white bread is perfectly safe and a good part of a normal, balanced diet. Why? In such a diet, you would obtain fiber from many other sources, notably fruits and vegetables.

In addition to fiber, other foods and nutrients too numerous to name here have been credited with dramatic curative powers they simply do not possess. Iodide, for instance, does nothing to cure baldness in men, and vitamin E is useless as a treatment to restore sexual potency.

The beef about beef

Are hormones in beef dangerous?

Counterbalancing the mania for "good foods" is the unnecessary avoidance of perfectly acceptable food products because certain advocates cast them as "bad."

American meat products, for instance, are often singled out for the "bad food" label—in part because of recent conflicts with the Europeans over processing methods. The argument goes that if the Europeans are refusing our meat products on the grounds that producers use hormones to promote growth, something must be terribly wrong with American meat!

Why are hormones used in cattle?

For the record, hormones are used to regulate the growth of livestock, to make the feed the animals eat work more efficiently, and to make the meat more tender. They are absolutely safe when properly used and contribute significantly to the high quality of our country's meat products.

Actually, the conflict over hormone treatments in beef is purely a trade issue, not a food safety issue. The objections of the Europeans, in actuality, are not health-based; rather they have to do with competition between European and American markets. The arguments about hormone treatments now look suspiciously like a convenient "cover" for use by the American and European media.

The conflict over American meat products arose as a result of an organized effort to keep American beef out of Europe, not because of any new clinical data suggesting that the products in question presented any danger. Quite to the contrary, there are no demonstrated health risks attributable to the use of hormones in beef cattle. Hormones are withdrawn from cattle well before the animal is slaughtered; there are only insignificant traces of hormones (if any) in the muscles and other tissues. Of course, the meat we eat is subject to rigorous inspection by the United States Department of Agriculture, as is poultry.

The final word on the hormone scare is: relax. American meat products are of extremely high quality. Those who advocate avoiding them because of alleged dangers associated with current processing methods have simply not studied the issue closely enough.

The water we drink

A similarly irrational approach is often taken in discussing another completely safe "consumable"—our drinking water.

Is fluoridation of water dangerous?

Fluoride added to drinking water at one part per million dramatically decreases dental caries (or cavities) and has no toxic effects. Yet many suggest that municipal water supplies are "impure" or "overprocessed" (they are neither, though the bottled water companies will not mind if you think they are) and that fluoride is somehow harmful to the communities that use it.

The continuing resistance to water fluoridation is inexplicable. As of this writing, only fifty percent of our water supply is fluoridated, meaning that half of our population is taking unnecessary dental health risks. Considering that dental cavities represent the most common of all diseases, this is extremely troublesome. (Incidentally, fluoride may also help prevent the development of osteoporosis, a painful and increasingly common disease among older people.)

Fluoridation of public water supplies is a safe, extremely effective means of preventing tooth decay. Its benefits and safety have been proven in study after study, but many people nevertheless believe it is dangerous or that it is a carcinogen. It is neither.

The trend today is toward "all-natural" water—witness the explosive growth of commercially available "spring waters." These waters, of course, are not fluoridated. As a result, they can be said to be less beneficial, from a health standpoint, than fluoridated tap water. Many of us are simply skeptical about "added chemicals" in our water or don't trust the authorities to fluoridate correctly. The fact remains, though, that fluoridation is a major weapon in the battle against tooth decay.

The only reason the practice of fluoridation is not more widespread seems to be that of paranoia.

Cholesterol

Of course, the most notorious recipient of the "bad food" label in today's society is probably dietary cholesterol. Many people regard it as a poison. Later in this book, we'll look at the complicated relationship between what we eat, our blood cholesterol levels, and the attendant risks to health.

Cashing in on the "good food, bad food" myth

It is no surprise to learn that certain companies are perfectly willing and able to take advantage of misperceptions people have about their food. The primary offender here is the health food industry, a large and growing sector of the economy that seems, sometimes, to operate on the principle that the less people know about food, the more likely they are to pay an exorbitant price for it.

Today's consumer is buffeted with confusing, often contradictory reports on pesticides, food processing methods, the virtues of vegetarian or macrobiotic diets, and the "overprocessing" of most commercially available foods. Health foods are often presented as a logical—if somewhat expensive—alternative.

How healthy *is* health food? We'll find out in the next chapter.

Chapter Three: How Healthy Are Health Foods?

The panic for organic

How dangerous are additives and pesticides in foods?

There is a myth promulgated by extremists that a modern industrialized society can somehow feed its population without using compounds designed to combat infestation in agricultural settings. Clearly, this is not so. Humans compete with insects for food. Considering the mass scale on which our food supply is produced, it is simply impossible to provide the public extremely large amounts of safe, high-quality food without using the weapons science has developed to counteract vermin.

How do foods sold in health food stores differ from those sold in supermarkets?

It's worth noting that additive- and pesticide-free "organic foods" (a meaningless term, by the way, since "organic" means only that the food contains carbon) can present a number of disadvantages from the consumer's standpoint. Such products typically deliver no additional health or nutritive value, look less attractive, and (for some types of food) spoil more quickly than their conventionally produced counterparts. What health food enthusiasts consider "natural" food is, all too often, food produced without the benefit of important quality control standards developed over the years.

The most significant difference between "supermarket food" and "health food" is price. For no demonstrated nutritional benefit, you'll often pay 50 to 75 percent more for a given type of product in a health food store than in a standard retail food outlet.

Do health foods present any potential dangers?

Products sold in health food stores often need more care than foods purchased in the supermarket, though the consumer is not always informed of this. Consider, for the purposes of illustrating the potential health risks, "natural" peanut butter. This is, typically, peanut butter that does not use an emulsifier, a harmless chemical additive that keeps the oil in the product from separating and rising to the top of the jar. Without the emulsifier, the peanut butter must be refrigerated. Often, however, consumers will leave the product on a counter or pantry shelf for days or weeks—resulting in the formation of rancid oil that may be stirred in later and consumed.

A popular marketing theme in health food stores is to promote "additive-free" foods. Many of these products, such as breads, tend to have problems with mold. This is not surprising, since foods with no preservatives must, like conventional products, sit in a warehouse for significant periods of time, or be transported from one point to another, giving mold plenty of time to flourish. Some molds, such as *Aspergillus flavus*, carry powerful carcinogens.

Most people think of food additives as being simply cosmetic. There certainly is some use in this area, though even cosmetic values are important. People must like the way food looks before they will eat it. Bruised, spotted, unattractive fruit is usually not bought in the first place—rendering the issue of its nutritional value meaningless.

What role do additives play in our foods?

Most food additives act as preservatives. They ensure the integrity of the food and they serve a necessary function in the enormous undertaking of feeding millions of people safely every day.

Food is a dynamic substance. It changes with time. You can get sick if you consume food that has been improperly processed or handled. Over the past decades, our society has developed extremely effective methods for dealing with the challenges presented by the mammoth task of handling and distributing our food. In the final analysis, food additives and other forms of technology, contrary to popular belief, usually represent the solution rather than the problem. It is far more significant, for instance, that an apple is free of mold growth (due in no small measure to the use of growth regulating chemicals) than that it contains barely measurable levels of Alar. And it is far more significant that a loaf of bread is free from other potentially harmful growths than that it contains small amounts of a harmless preservative.

Indeed, far from presenting any public health problem, our use of food additives such as antioxidants, found in many cereal and bread products, may contribute to our country's comparatively low rate of stomach cancer!

When the task is to meet the nutritional needs of a society of 250 million people, pesticides, additives, and preservatives represent essential tools, not hazards. Without these elements, we would quickly be faced with a diminished food supply of poor quality, available only at extremely high prices.

Are food additives necessary?

Health food store "doctors"

Rightly or wrongly, people expect more from health foods than they do from foods they buy in a supermarket. Because these stores, like supermarkets, are businesses (and often, like supermarkets, very *large* businesses) operated for profit, there is pressure to deliver what the customer wants. Often, however, health food outlets cross the line between enthusiastic marketing and overt misrepresentation about the health benefits of products they sell.

Many of the employees of these establishments make claims in person for given products that manufacturers are prohibited by law from placing on the packaging! It's quite common for a health food "expert" to "prescribe" vitamin E for impotence, or pantothenic acid (one of the B-complex vitamins) for baldness, or Laetrile (falsely called vitamin B_{17}) for the treatment of cancer, as well as scores of other dubious remedies.

Beyond the problems of product misrepresentation and fraud, there is the very real danger of actual disease being "misdiagnosed" by these would-be doctors. Practicing medicine without a license is illegal. In our view, however, medicine is widely practiced across the counters of the nation's health food stores, at considerable risk to the "patients."

If you think you have a health problem of any kind, *don't* trust the person at the health food store checkout counter to understand it or be able to suggest a remedy. See your doctor.

What is a macrobiotic diet?

The dangers of macrobiotic dieting

One notable fad that gained popularity in the 1970s (though it now seems to have waned) is the macrobiotic movement. The philosophies associated with this movement—and its attendant dietary regimen—are still closely associated with many of the "New Age" groups.

Some years back, a Japanese philosopher by the name of Georges Osawa formulated what eventually became known as the Zen Macrobiotic Diet. This diet consisted of various stages; the more advanced one's spiritual development, the further up the macrobiotic "ladder" one moved.

What is the Zen Macrobiotic Diet?

The first two stages presented no problem, but severe malnutrition awaited those who "progressed" to the final levels. The later stages eliminated various foods without any consideration for compensating for the loss of important nutrients. Finally, the most "advanced" followers of this regimen were instructed to consume *only brown rice,* supplemented with very little liquid, for protracted periods. It is not surprising that a number of deaths were reported among those who followed this senseless diet to its lethal conclusion.

Fortunately, the Zen Macrobiotic Diet has passed from the scene, though new macrobiotic diets have surfaced. The latest versions do not carry the same risks as Osawa's inept regimen, but they offer no measurable health advantages over a standard, balanced diet—and they're not much fun to eat, either.

Some of the exaggerations and distortions associated with macrobiotic diets have gained wide acceptance. For instance, many have been led to believe by macrobiotic enthusiasts that animal proteins "cause putrefaction in the stomach." Actually, amino acids are not broken down in the stomach, but they can be broken down to amines in the bowel. These amines are then excreted safely in the urine. The same thing happens when the amino acids are of vegetable origin.

Can macrobiotic diets cure cancer?

Some years ago, a doctor received wide media attention for having "cured" his cancer with a macrobiotic diet. (We must remember, of course, that some cancers do go into remission with or without such a diet.) Though his claims were received with great skepticism by much of the medical community, that was not the part of the story many people wanted to hear—and, for the most part, it was not what people were told.

The most prominent current macrobiotic guidelines have been promulgated by one Michio Kushi, founder of the Kushi Institute, the East-West Foundation, and the Erewhon Natural Foods Company. According to Kushi, macrobiotic diets and philosophies represent religion that isn't religion and medicine that isn't medicine, all based on "native and intuitive common sense." What this boils down to is that Kushi is another in a long series of quasi-mystic food faddists. The diet follows these guidelines:

> *50 percent or more whole grains and their products*
> *10 to 15 percent beans, seeds, and their products*
> *15 percent or less animal food (fish and seafood only)*
> *Occasional fruit in small volumes*
> *Fermented food (such as soy sauce, pickles, wine, or beer) in small volumes*

Kushi's macrobiotic diet excludes meat, poultry, dairy foods, tropical fruits, soft drinks, coffee, sugar, honey, syrups, foods with preservatives or additives, refined grains, hot spices, and a category described as "mass-produced industrialized foods."

What there is left to eat must be chewed fifty times or more per mouthful.

From a nutritional standpoint, such diets are unnecessarily restrictive, though certainly not as dangerous as the Zen diet forwarded by Osawa. The main health benefits that can be ascribed to most diets based on food faddism are attributable to the placebo effect and not to any magic associated with chewing mouthfuls of sunflower seeds for hours on end.

Vegetarians and vegans

What about vegetarian diets?

Most vegetarian diets—the ones that include dairy products and eggs—present no problems if sensibly planned. One must, however, be very careful with a strict vegetarian, or vegan, diet. This regimen excludes all animal products from a person's menu: no fish, no chicken, no eggs, no milk, and, for the stricter groups, no honey.

What are the dangers of removing all animal products from the diet?

Nutritional difficulties arise in these diets, in part because vitamin B_{12} is an essential nutrient—a nutrient found only in products of animal origin. When people exclude all animal products from their diet, they must take supplements (often through injections) to be sure they're meeting their nutritional needs. Special emphasis is laid here on the question of meeting the needs of young children, some of whom may not react well to lesser degrees of vegetarianism, much less the removal of all animal products from the diet.

Ensuring adequate consumption of vitamin B_{12} is not the only problem facing those who wish to follow a vegan diet. Calcium and phosphorus, nutrients usually provided by the dairy group, must also be taken into account. These two nutrients work together to form and maintain our bones and teeth; the degree to which both are present in the diet is important. (The Recommended Dietary Allowances for calcium and phosphorus for those over age eighteen are 800 milligrams of each per day.) Removing dairy products from one's meal plan eliminates important sources of calcium and phosphorus.

Fortunately, there are alternative sources of calcium and phosphorus available to those who wish to limit or restrict the intake of dairy products. The main options are summarized below.

How can vegans eat a balanced diet?

(By the way, these alternate sources often work equally well for individuals who are lactose intolerant. If you fall into this category, ask your doctor about the following foods if he or she has not already suggested them.)

Corn tortillas. A six-inch corn tortilla provides about a 1.5:1 ratio of calcium to phosphorus; the favorable ratio is 1:1 after the first year of life. In conjunction with other foods, corn tortillas should probably be included in a vegetarian or vegan diet and can contribute favorably to calcium and phosphorus intake levels. *Calcium per serving (one tortilla):* 60 mg. *Phosphorus per serving:* 42 mg.

Tofu and/or soybean milk. These products, while certainly not in the same league as cheese or skim or whole milk, can provide comparatively high amounts of calcium and phosphorus when compared with other nondairy foods. Soybean milk is a less impressive source of calcium than tofu, which typically provides the two minerals at the favorable 1:1 ratio. *Calcium per serving:* Tofu (3 1/2-oz. serving): 128 mg. Soy milk (1 cup serving): 55 mg. *Phosphorus per serving:* Tofu (3 1/2-oz. serving): 126 mg. Soy milk (1 cup serving): 126 mg.

Greens and broccoli. Cooked broccoli offers a calcium-to-phosphorus ratio similar to that of corn tortillas; collard greens are notably lighter in phosphorus, with a ratio of almost 5:1. In nonvegetarian diets one might suggest a slice of meat alongside the greens; a serving of cooked pinto beans, however, would serve the same purpose. *Calcium per serving:* Broccoli (1 stalk): 160 mg.

Collard greens (1 cup): 360 mg. *Phosphorus per serving:* Broccoli (1 stalk): 110 mg. Collard greens (1 cup): 100 mg.

Note: The above is based on the recommended intake of calcium and phosphorus for all persons *except infants one year of age or younger.* For this group, the ratio of calcium to phosphorus should be higher—1.5:1.

In addition to vitamin B_{12}, calcium, and phosphorus, another nutrient can be underconsumed in some vegetarian diets: niacin. Niacin levels in plants are low; vegans must consume very large amounts of legumes (such as pinto beans or green peas) to compensate. (By way of example, note that the Recommended Dietary Allowance for a male between 19 and 22 is 19 milligrams of niacin equivalent—and that a cup of cooked peas provides only 1.8 milligrams.)

A few additional words of caution are in order about vegan diets when compared with vegetarian diets that include eggs and dairy products. Zinc and iron deficiencies are common problems for those who follow the vegan diet, and while some common vegetarian foods (such as spinach) are good sources of iron, zinc can be trickier to obtain in adequate amounts unless the diet is planned with great care. (Three cups of cooked green peas or the equivalent are necessary to meet the daily zinc needs of an adult male.) In addition, vegans must be sure that a mixture of protein sources (legumes and nuts, legumes and cereals, cereals and nuts, or all three simultaneously) are present at *every meal*—otherwise problems with protein nutrition may develop.

If adequate precautions are taken, the vegan and vegetarian diets can be satisfactory. These precautions, however, among other consequences of the health food movement, necessitate dietary scrutiny that, in our view, entails more inconvenience, discomfort, and sacrifice than it's worth.

Chapter Four: Is Our Food Safe?

Bad apples?

Should I worry about Alar residues in apples?

The recent media-fueled panic about apples "poisoned" by trace residues of Alar stands out as one of the more overblown diet-related episodes in recent memory. The Alar scare can serve as a good introduction to the emotionally charged issue of food safety in America.

Meryl Streep, whose celebrity appearances played a major role in bringing this issue to national attention, is admittedly an excellent actress. She turns out, however, to be an inept and ill-informed toxicologist. Those who are interested in learning the facts are advised to give greater heed to the opinions of the many scientists and health professionals who have spent entire careers in the relevant fields. A summary of the facts surrounding the Alar scare follows.

How do we know if carcinogens are in food?

What causes cancer?

There was a time about 30 years ago when many cancers were thought to have been caused by chemicals in the general environment. Although it was firmly established by the late 1950s that cigarette smoking was the leading preventable cause of cancer in the United States, the scientific community, understandably, wanted to reduce cancer further, and believed that all that was necessary was to identify certain cancer-causing chemicals and eliminate them. It was also thought that those chemicals emanated strictly from industrial sources. Accordingly, scientists tested only chemicals that were manmade.

The chosen means of testing these chemicals was through animal studies—in other words, feeding large amounts of the chemicals to laboratory animals. If the animals developed cancer at a rate higher than expected, the assumption was that people ingesting much smaller amounts would too.

The objective, then, was a clear one: get rid of any measurable amounts of the chemicals that caused cancer in the laboratory, and the population would be healthier. Over the next few decades, however, a number of new developments changed the landscape dramatically.

Do minute amounts of carcinogens in a normal diet play a major role in health risks?

First, of course, the technology advanced. Today, we can detect levels of chemicals that were completely undetectable thirty years ago. And we now realize that the mere presence of trace levels of a substance does not, by definition, demonstrate a health hazard. Specifically, such trace levels do not necessarily reflect any increased risk of cancer.

Second, and more dramatic, was the realization that cancer-causing agents occur not only in synthetic sources, but also throughout nature. In other words, "carcinogens"—that is, chemicals that cause cancer in high doses in animals—are present throughout nature and therefore in our food supply.

This does not, by any stretch of the imagination, lead to the conclusion that most foods pose hazards. These natural carcinogens, like most synthetic ones, show up at barely measurable levels. All the discovery means is that the assumptions by which toxicologists worked in the 1950s and 1960s (namely, that nature was "carcinogen-free" and only synthetic chemicals suspect) were in error.

Are toxins and carcinogens in food the same as the ones in hazardous workplaces?

It is important to keep in mind that the naturally occurring carcinogens have little in common with the chemicals and other materials that have been linked with occupation-related cancer. These agents would include asbestos and vinyl chloride—substances to which, unlike natural carcinogens, a person would have to be subjected for long-term, *high-dose* exposures to assume a high risk of developing specific types of cancer. Nevertheless, in determining that cancer-causing agents are much more common than initially believed, scientists have concluded that the world abounds with carcinogens—of both natural and synthetic origin—at very low levels.

Furthermore, these trace levels play little or no role in causing human cancer in the developed world. Humans have a whole array of defenses against carcinogenic chemicals, particularly at low doses. This is not a surprising development, considering that we and our ancestors have been safely ingesting foods that contain carcinogens for millions of years!

(It is possible that naturally occurring carcinogens may pose a problem in less developed countries, where food quality and processing methods are inferior. Of course, living in such a country poses a great many health risks when compared with living in developed nations like the United States, England, or Sweden.)

The main point is that *finding* any carcinogen—manmade or naturally occurring—is not enough. Furthermore, the idea that most food could somehow be produced without trace levels of carcinogens or toxins is simply wrong. The *dose* of whatever chemical is being discussed, not its mere presence, is the key in determining if a health risk is present.

Are carcinogens found only in manmade materials?

Part of the problem is the terminology used to discuss the issue of "chemicals in foods." Most of us would probably choose, without hesitation, a dinner that is "free of chemicals" over one that "contains chemicals." That dinner, however, would have to be an empty plate! *All* food is composed of chemicals.

Take, for instance, a potato. A potato is a complex aggregate of at least 150 different chemicals, all put there by nature. Nature also put into the natural potato such "organic" niceties as arsenic, solanine, nitrate, and a number of other toxic chemicals—all of which could be extremely dangerous if you took them in high doses. But there is such a minute amount of these chemicals in each individual potato that ordinary quantities of potatoes are perfectly safe to eat. (For that matter, the same could be said for virtually any quantity you'd be able to consume that *wasn't* ordinary. In other words, you could certainly eat several dozen potatoes, or even several *bushels* of potatoes, without worry—though probably not without indigestion.)

We consider now the simple, all-American, standard-issue apple. It may contain near-unmeasurable amounts of a substance that can, at high doses, cause an increase of cancer in mice—namely Alar, a chemical used in the processing of low-cost, high-quality apples. Why, if we can justify eating a potato that contains arsenic, should consumers flee in terror from supermarkets stocking apples that contain comparable levels of Alar?

The seemingly objective, impassive media claim is that some apples "contain Alar, a substance that has been shown to cause cancer in laboratory animals." True enough. But, in the interests of fair play, should we not shine an equally harsh spotlight on the "recklessness" of the potato industry, which has been shipping out goods known to "contain arsenic" for decades?

How about the producers of table pepper, whose product is known to "contain safrole," a component that has been proven carcinogenic in massive doses to laboratory animals? And after the potato and condiment industries have been completely decimated, we can move on to celery and parsley, which contain psoralens, potent light-activated carcinogens.

With further research, tomatoes might follow in short order, and then strawberries. In no time at all, with hard work and a little dedication, we can completely cripple the agricultural and food-producing sectors, and be left with very few foods to eat.

"Dangerous" meals...?

On the following pages you'll find one of the most dramatic exemplifications of how important perspective is when discussing our food supply. We reproduce here a "Holiday Dinner Menu" showing just how "dangerous" common foods could be considered—if we held them to the same standards employed by those behind the Alar scare!

(The following excerpt is reprinted with the kind permission of the American Council on Science and Health.)

Excerpts From

"DOES NATURE KNOW BEST? NATURAL CARCINOGENS IN AMERICAN FOOD"

A publication of the American Council on Science and Health

Picture this: You glance at a newspaper and notice a headline announcing that laboratory tests have shown that a substance in our food supply is a carcinogen. You only see the headline; you don't have time to read the story. What type of substance would you guess that the carcinogen is?

If you guessed that it was a food additive, a pesticide, or some other type of man-made contaminant, you would have a very good chance of being right. For it is these types of chemicals, man-made substances added to food either accidentally, or deliberately, that make the headlines. However, there is another large group of carcinogenic chemicals that has attracted little attention as yet: naturally occurring carcinogenic substances in food. These natural carcinogens are in fact much more widespread and numerous than the man-made carcinogens in food and are present in much larger amounts.

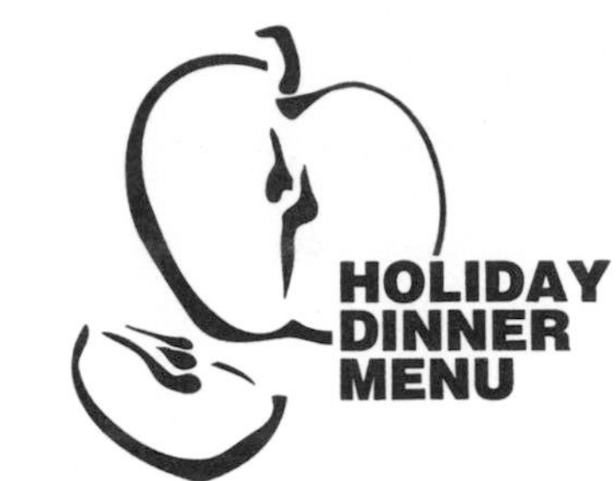

WHAT'S ON THE PLATE	*WHAT'S IN IT**
	APPETIZERS
CREAM OF MUSHROOM SOUP	hydrazines
	FRESH VEGETABLE TRAY
CARROTS	carotatoxin, myristicin, isoflavones, nitrate
RADISHES	glucosinolates, nitrate
CHERRY TOMATOES	hydrogen peroxide, nitrate, quercetin glycoside, tomatine
CELERY	nitrate, psoralens
	ENTREES
ROAST TURKEY	heterocyclic amines, malonaldehyde
BREAD STUFFING *(with onions, celery, black pepper and mushrooms)*	benzo(a)pyrene, di- and tri-sulfides ethyl carbamate, furan derivatives dihydrazines, psoralens, safrole
CRANBERRY SAUCE	eugenol, furan derivatives

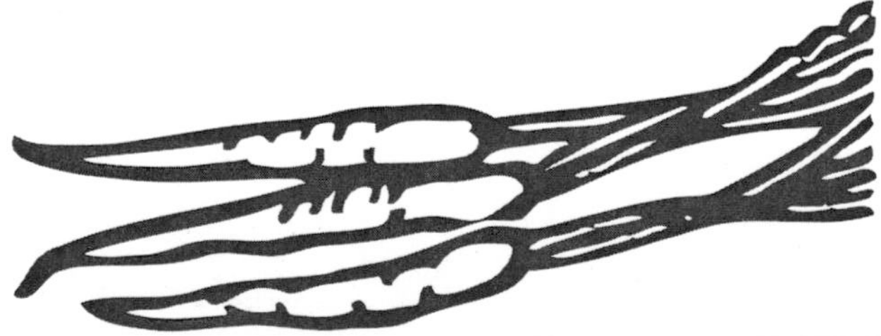

CHOICE OF VEGETABLE

LIMA BEANS	cyanogenetic glycosides
BROCCOLI SPEARS	allyl isothiocyanate, glucosinolates, goitrin, nitrate
BAKED POTATO	amylase inhibitors, arsenic, chaconine, isoflavones, nitrate, oxalic acid, solanine
SWEET POTATO	cyanogenetic glycosides, furan derivatives, nitrate
ROLLS	amylase inhibitors, benzo(a)pyrene, ethyl carbamate, furan derivatives, diacetyl

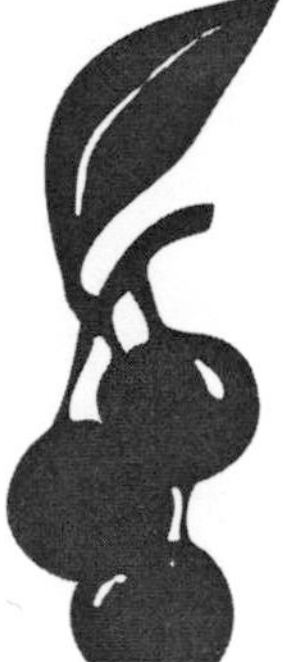

DESSERTS

PUMPKIN PIE	myristicin, nitrate, safrole
APPLE PIE	acetaldehyde, isoflavones, phlorizin, quercetin glycoside, safrole

BEVERAGES

COFFEE	benzy(a)pyrene, caffeine, chlorogenic acid, hydrogen peroxide, methylglyoxal, tannins
TEA	benzo(a)pyrene, caffeine, quercetin glycosides, tannins
RED WINE	alcohol, ethyl carbamate, methylglyoxal, tannins, tyramine
WATER	nitrate

ASSORTED NUTS

MIXED NUTS	aflatoxins

* See toxicological summary on following page to review health effects of high-dose exposure to these natural chemicals.

Menu analysis prepared by ACSH staff and its Directors and Scientific Advisors, with technical assistance from Leonard T. Flynn, Ph.D., M.B.A., a scientific consultant.

TOXIC EFFECTS OF HIGH DOSES OF NATURALLY OCCURRING CHEMICALS THAT NORMALLY ARE HARMLESS IN THE AMOUNTS USUALLY FOUND IN FOODS AND BEVERAGES

ACETALDEHYDE (apples) - mutagen in short-term biological test systems (for example, the Ames test) and animal carcinogen.
AFLATOXINS (nuts) - can induce toxic effects in humans and are among the most potent mutagens and animal carcinogens known.
ALCOHOL (wine) - human carcinogen and teratogen (can cause birth defects).
ALLYL ISOTHIOCYANATE (broccoli) - animal carcinogen.
AMYLASE INHIBITORS (potatoes, rolls) - interfere with animal and human digestive enzyme systems.
ARSENIC (potatoes) - human carcinogen and toxic effects observed in humans.
BENZO(A)PYRENE (bread, rolls, coffee, tea) - animal carcinogen.
CAFFEINE (coffee, tea) - human toxin and animal teratogen.
CAROTATOXIN (carrots) - nerve poison in animals.
CHACONINE (potatoes) - toxic alkaloid that can strongly inhibit human nerve transmission (cholinesterase inhibitor).
CHLOROGENIC ACID (coffee) - bacterial mutagen.
CYANOGENETIC GLYCOSIDES (lima beans, sweet potatoes, apples) - when chewed or ingested can release cyanide, a human toxin.
DIACETYL (butter, coffee) - bacterial mutagen.
DI- AND TRI-SULFIDES (onions) - antithyroid activity in animals (see glucosinolates).
ETHYL CARBAMATE (bread, rolls, wine) - animal carcinogen.
EUGENOL (cranberry sauce) - animal carcinogen.
FURAN DERIVATIVES (bread, onions, celery, mushrooms, sweet potatoes, rolls, cranberry sauce) - many are mutagens in test systems.
GLUCOSINOLATES (broccoli, radishes) - interfere with use of iodine (antithyroid activity) causing thyroid enlargement (goiter) in humans.
GOITRIN (broccoli) - antithyroid compound in humans (see glucosinolates).
HETEROCYCLIC AMINES (turkey) - many are mutagens in test systems.
HYDRAZINES (mushrooms) - many are animal carcinogens.
HYDROGEN PEROXIDE (coffee, tomatoes) - mutagen in test systems and animal carcinogen.
ISOFLAVONES (apples, carrots, potatoes) - have estrogenic effect (mimic female sex hormone activity) in animals.
MALONALDEHYDE (turkey) - mutagenic in test systems.
METHYLGLYOXAL (coffee, wine) - animal carcinogen and bacterial mutagen.
MYRISTICIN (carrots, black pepper, nutmeg) - human hallucinogen.
NITRATE (broccoli, carrots, celery, radishes, tomatoes, potatoes, pumpkins, water) - toxic in humans; can also convert to nitrite and subsequently form nitrosamines (animal carcinogens).
OXALIC ACID (potatoes) - human toxin which can form kidney stones.
PHLORIZIN (apples) - interferes with cell enzyme systems in animals.
PSORALENS (celery) - human mutagens and carcinogens.
QUERCETIN GLYCOSIDES (tomatoes, apples, tea) - quercetin is an animal carcinogen and mutagen in bacteria and insects.
SAFROLE (nutmeg, cinnamon, black pepper) - animal carcinogen.
SOLANINE (potatoes) - alkaloid that can strongly inhibit human nerve transmission (cholinesterase inhibitor). Can also cause gastrointestinal tract irritation (abdominal pain, diarrhea, or ulceration).
TANNINS (wine, coffee, tea) - animal carcinogens. Can interfere with human nutrition, and cause growth depression and intestinal damage.
TOMATINE (tomatoes) - interferes with nerve transmission in humans (cholinesterase inhibitor).
TYRAMINE (wine) - can cause blood pressure elevation in some humans.

If an apple a day keeps the doctor away—what will a truckload do?

How many apples would you have to eat to approximate the levels associated with increased cancer in animals?

Eating apples—even those treated with the much-maligned Alar—as part of a normal diet poses no health risk for the general population.

To get an idea of the level of exaggeration implicit in the absurd idea that apples are "bad for" anyone—specifically including young children—consider this. If you wanted to duplicate, on a human scale, the results that identify Alar as a cancer-causing agent, you would have to consume quantities equivalent to those given by scientists to mice in laboratories. What, exactly, would that entail?

You would have to sit down, muster up, in the interests of science, all the willpower at your disposal, and eat a great many apples.

How many apples would you have to eat?

Five hundred pounds. At one sitting.

It doesn't take a Ph.D. in toxicology to determine that, in eating such ludicrously large amounts, you'd probably expire—but not from cancer!

Three important facts

Didn't CONSUMER REPORTS say apples with Alar are dangerous?

There are three key points that have been ignored or glossed over in most discussions about Alar.

1) The extremely high Alar doses fed to mice simply cannot be duplicated in a standard human diet.

2) Current levels of Alar found in apples (if, indeed, any can be found at all) fall well below long-established government guidelines.

3) Alar has been used *since 1967* without a single case of cancer or any other disease attributed to its consumption at approved trace levels in apples.

Though these points are well established and accepted throughout the scientific community, they seem to matter not a whit to the nation's newspapers, television stations, and radio talk show hosts. Even as respected an outlet as *Consumer Reports* has focused only on the fact that highly sophisticated techniques could detect Alar, totally ignoring the fact that no person, anywhere, could be expected to consume enough of the Alar "present" to cause cancer.

The emotionally loaded issue of "carcinogens in the nation's food supply" makes great copy. But the copy never addresses the fact that Alar itself presents no demonstrable health risk and has been used safely for over two decades. Furthermore, it ignores the broader reality that *carcinogens at trace levels abound in natural foods.*

But what does that matter? If you can get the words "cancer," "apples," and "children" in the same lead sentence, nobody's going to bother to read the rest of the article anyway. Better to stay with the human drama, the compelling notion that the apple growers of America have been slowly poisoning us and our children for years. If the facts get in the way, set them aside. These, apparently, are the standards for some (but fortunately, not all) of today's journalists.

Should agricultural chemicals be banned?

Shouldn't Alar and other agricultural compounds be banned—to "play it safe?"

Given the omnipresence of naturally occurring chemicals that cause cancer in animals, banning something like Alar is like removing a grain of sand from the beach. Such a ban would have no positive impact on public health—though it would certainly dramatically raise the prices paid by consumers for apples.

Such unpleasant developments may well be in the cards. As this book goes to press, the manufacturer of Alar, Uniroyal, is expected to withdraw the product from the domestic market—more as a reaction to pressure generated by news reports than from a review of any new scientific findings.

Let's address for a moment the reasoning that if there is even the tiniest, barely measurable chance that it could affect a child, if it causes cancer in a mouse in any dosage whatsoever, Alar (or any other chemical that can cause cancer in mice) should not be used.

It should be clear enough by now that if we follow this standard, we will have virtually no food left on the shelves of any store in the United States. Practically speaking, certain components (or chemicals, if you prefer) of every product would fail the test, and hundreds upon hundreds of harmless products would have to be removed from the market. Why? Roughly two thirds of all the chemicals tested on laboratory animals are eventually classified as carcinogens. In addition, we must remember, such overreaction could mean that the country's farmers would be left without many of the tools necessary to produce what we eat.

Why use agricultural chemicals?

The food industry doesn't go to the trouble, time, and considerable expense of using agricultural chemicals for the fun of it. The compounds are used for a reason, and there are considerable health risks associated with the often-posed suggestion of banning them outright.

The general public is told, for instance, that Alar is used to make apples crunchier and improve their color. It has those cosmetic effects, but actually, Alar is used primarily to keep apples on the tree longer, so that they all fall at the same time. If the apples fall unevenly, the apples stay on the ground too long and rot. Insects lay their eggs in the rotting apples and insect infestation results.

This is not to say that if Alar were banned we would all have to resort to eating insect-infested apples. The food industry would find other ways to deal with the insect problem—but those other ways would probably mean higher prices for the consumer, lower quality, and less selection and convenience than we've become accustomed to.

Considering that not a single case of human cancer has ever been attributed to Alar despite widespread use dating back to the Johnson Administration, why should consumers be asked to make such sacrifices? Similarly, if we cannot hold all food producers to the standards being imposed on apple growers—and in the view of the authors, we clearly cannot—what, specifically, is gained by throwing the agricultural economies of the apple-producing New England and Pacific Northwest regions into total chaos?

The bicycle ride

Some members of the news media seem intent on distracting people from real risks because illusory ones are more interesting. And for the most part, no one seems to mind.

A woman we know, upon hearing the first wave of the Alar scare stories, threw away perhaps thirty dollars worth of apples, applesauce, and apple butter from her pantry. She was unwilling, she explained, to expose her daughter to "any risk, no matter how slight."

The next morning, she was seen riding her bicycle down a steep, rocky road into town. Her daughter, smiling happily, was seated precariously on the back of the bike. Neither the little girl nor the mother was wearing a helmet—leaving both at risk for serious head injury. One wonders about people's priorities.

The great American food scare: a market phenomenon, not a medical alert

As the Alar episode suggests, many of the charges regarding the safety of our food supply have more adrenaline than evidence fueling them.

The facts, as we'll see, indicate that the American food supply is the safest on the face of the earth. Nevertheless, from time to time, health-food zealots and other sensationalists seem intent on frightening people out of their wits. The Alar scare, after all, isn't the only story that's been blown out of proportion.

When food panics surface, the consequences usually have more to do with economics than with public health. And the irony of it all is that many short-lived scares are eventually ignored completely by the public!

It is usually thought that Americans will not tolerate any type of manmade carcinogen in their diets. However, it's become increasingly clear that, if there is a perceived need for a product, Americans are usually willing to use it—regardless of the bad press it may receive.

The saccharin ban

How dangerous is saccharin?

For example, in March 1977 the Food and Drug Administration announced that it was going to ban saccharin. The reason: saccharin was shown to cause bladder cancer in laboratory animals in a two-generation Canadian study.

Consumers, however, were furious that the government planned to take away their saccharin—at that point, their only available low-calorie sweetener. Saccharin users, it turned out, represented a sizeable portion of the public. Consequently, Congress passed override legislation, and the announced ban never occurred. (Instead, a warning label was mandated.)

Saccharin, of course, is perfectly safe in quantities people (rather than rats) consume. We use the sweetener widely today—in coffee, sodas, and even in toothpaste—with no ill effect whatsoever. Saccharin has been used since early in this century, and studies of diabetics (who use substantial amounts of it compared with the rest of the population) show no unusual cancer patterns linked to the use of the sweetener. Nevertheless, saccharin is a "carcinogen" in the same way Alar is—both can, at high doses, cause cancer in rodents. But there is no evidence that either poses a hazard to the health of humans at usual levels of consumption.

Why do Americans tolerate saccharin but fear Alar? Because saccharin is familiar and has a perceived benefit. Alar, on the other hand, is invisible and unknown—and thus presents an emotional (rather than a medical) risk.

As we have seen, simply attaching the word "carcinogen" to a given chemical does not convey enough information—and it does not, over the long term, necessarily mean a product will (or should!) be withdrawn from the market. In the meantime, however, there will be a great deal of unnecessary panic and pointless economic disruption at the height of the scare.

Certainly, if you read a news report that a food "contains a carcinogen," you should probably get more information before you start tossing the product from your refrigerator. Remember, there are some carcinogens people decide to tolerate—with no harmful effects!—because they have a genuine desire for the products that contain them. Apples, like saccharin, will probably weather the storm. (For the record, Americans consume much more saccharin than Alar, but, as we've seen, Alar has been framed as a more emotional issue.)

We should remember that the food industry will react to what the market demands. The industry always works to give consumers what they want, not, as some people would believe, to give them foods laced with hazardous chemicals. Why, after all, would food producers go to the trouble of poisoning their market base?

Is palm oil dangerous?

That's the question a lot of Americans had on their minds when they read about yet another ingredient in our food products alleged to have harmful effects: tropical oils such as palm oil. These are used as shortening in many processed foods. Thanks to a maverick media campaign by a single disgruntled consumer, more misinformation was spread in a shorter period of time on this topic than we have space to address here.

The "controversy," such as it is, centers on the saturated fat level of the tropical oils—which range from 49 to 80 percent, admittedly fairly high. Consumption of saturated fat has been shown to raise blood cholesterol levels in some (not all) individuals. That was enough! Tropical oils—and the foods containing them—were dubbed "poison" overnight.

Never mind that the actual level of consumption of these oils is by no means high. (They account for only one to two percent of total calories in the American diet and are negligible in terms of their effect on average total fat intake.) Never mind that the amounts of saturated fat contained in the crackers, cookies, and other products in question were, in the context of a full day's diet, of marginal importance when compared with other foods. And never mind that half of all adults register no change whatsoever in their serum cholesterol levels through dietary changes! Saturated fat was "poison," tropical oils had saturated fat, and food manufacturers were lacing our foods with tropical oils. Therefore the food industry wanted to poison us!

Needless to say, the reaction from the industry was swift and decisive. New formulations were announced, new packages were designed, new ad campaigns launched. The perception of risk—rather than risk itself—carried the day.

Food producers, in essence, do what the shopper tells them. They will, generally speaking, market products in whatever way sells the most units. They will even misrepresent science, if that is what people want. The objective, though, is not so much to deceive as it is to label products in a way that will appease the consumer. Experience has shown these companies that the words "organic," "natural," "no palm oil," "cholesterol-free," and a host of similar terms can greatly influence customers, even though foods that carry such labels are not necessarily better for one's health.

It's probably fair to say that in pursuing such tactics the food industry is contributing to its own problems. In many ways, it's not that surprising that some have lost faith in the food industry, which presently is more interested in short-term sales than it is in long-term commitments to scientifically sound food information.

Has the American diet been stripped of most of its nutrients through processing?

The "overprocessing" myth

Beyond the argument that modern food processing techniques add "harmful chemicals" or "poisons" to the average American's diet lies a more nebulous claim. This is the idea repeatedly put forward by health food enthusiasts that nutrients are "bleached out" of foods, leading to a generally poorer quality of nutrition.

Exactly the opposite is true.

Americans have the most fortified food supply in the world. In large measure, this is attributable to the pioneering work done in the Roosevelt Administration during the Great Depression. It was during this period that the federal government initiated minimum standards for basic nutrients and mandated the fortification of much commercially produced food.

Nevertheless, it is a common complaint that food produced on a large scale, such as bread or cereal, is "overprocessed" and therefore less nutritious than "natural" foods.

Some people protest, for example, that in processing grains during the production of white bread, producers "strip vitamins" from the flour. The statement will usually end there. In reality, the major nutrients stripped during processing are restored before the processing is finished, and the minor ones not restored are readily obtained from other foods in the diet.

Real risks vs. imaginary risks

From a purely objective standpoint, and taking into account as many of the potential risks and benefits as possible, there is not and has never been another nation on earth with a better food supply that presents fewer health risks than that found in the United States of America.

What does that really mean to the person in the supermarket, curious about the safety of food about to be purchased? It means that if you could choose among all the societies and countries in human history, and you wanted the safest food supply possible, you could do no better than what we have now in the United States in the latter part of the twentieth century.

It usually comes as no surprise to Americans to learn that their food is generally safer and more wholesome than food purchased or prepared in, say, Senegal or Bangladesh. What is less well known is the fact that the American food production, processing, and supply methods are demonstrably superior to those found in some highly industrialized regions such as Western Europe!

Even in that part of the world you'll encounter, for instance, improper packaging, questionable mass production methods, and unacceptable hygiene practices on the retail level.

Is the American food supply safe?

There is no question that the American diet and the processing methods that make it possible are the best anywhere. Foods that do not take advantage of current technology and production advances are no more "wholesome" than conventional foods.

Does that mean that there are no dangers associated with the foods you can buy in the supermarket? Far from it. However, because we live in a technologically advanced society, we can turn our attention to the one area where there remains some genuine risk with regard to the food we eat—how it's prepared in our homes.

What food risks are associated with handling and preparation?

In the United States, most problems relating to food safety generally occur once the food is in your kitchen. Fortunately, these risks can be virtually eliminated once one understands the basics of food hygiene.

For instance, it may seem innocent enough to make hamburger patties and then toss a salad without washing your hands. However, anything that is not cooked, like a salad, will bear the bacteria from the raw meat that touches it. This is a good way to court unnecessary health risks.

Another example: say you go to a barbecue and you see the host bring out raw chicken on a platter before placing the bird on the grill. An hour later, he puts the cooked chicken on the same platter. Of course, the platter has been exposed to bacteria from the raw chicken. Food should always be served from clean dishes and utensils.

Beyond such basic precautions, however, there's no reason for concern about the safety of our food. One wonders, though, about the possible adverse effects of spending night and day worrying about it!

SECTION TWO: CHOLESTEROL IN PERSPECTIVE

Chapter Five: What Is Cholesterol?

What is cholesterol?

Ask the average American what cholesterol is and you are likely to hear something like, "It's something in hamburgers and sausages that's bad for you." With all the media attention over the last several years, the word "cholesterol" has simply become a catch-word supposed (erroneously) to be synonymous with coronary heart disease. In reality, cholesterol itself does not directly cause any heart disease.

Cholesterol is a white, waxy, fatty substance found in virtually all foods derived from animal sources;

it is an intrinsic part of animal tissues. It is found in hamburgers and roast chicken, in cheese sandwiches and fish, in scrambled eggs and buttered toast, and in beef stew and chicken noodle soup. It is also found in our bodies, whether we eat animal foods or not, and this is fortunate, since our bodies couldn't function without it.

Where does the cholesterol in our bodies come from?

Most of our cholesterol is manufactured in our bodies. For example, an adult manufactures about one gram (1,000 milligrams, or mg) of cholesterol each day, in addition to the cholesterol consumed from foods. As a result, most of the cholesterol present in the bloodstream is produced every day by synthesis, chiefly by the liver.

Many people consider the consumption of cholesterol, in and of itself, to be a health hazard. This is not the case. The risks associated with cholesterol intake have been vastly overstated by the media and even by some public health officials.

The cholesterol in our bodies is essential for good health. It is a naturally present substance that our bodies need in order to function properly, not a poison you ingest from the "wrong" foods. It is required for the transport of fat in the blood, for the manufacture of bile acids needed to absorb fats, for successful pregnancy and resistance to stress, for the maintenance of functional and water-resistant skin, and as a precursor for the synthesis of male and female sex hormones.

Furthermore, cholesterol is a component of every membrane in the body. The widespread perception, then, that the presence of cholesterol in the human body is somehow intrinsically harmful is a distortion of the truth.

There is on record the case of a child with a hereditary inability to produce adequate amounts of cholesterol. At two years of age the child was hospitalized because of serious developmental problems, mental retardation, and cataracts. His serum cholesterol level was approximately fifty percent lower than one would expect to find in a healthy male child of the same age. Analysis of his tissues showed the absence of a certain enzyme needed in cholesterol synthesis. Unfortunately, before his doctor could initiate treatment with cholesterol, the child died of infection and failure of his tissues to maintain normal metabolism.

Dietary cholesterol

How much dietary cholesterol do Americans consume?

The average American consumes 400 mg of dietary cholesterol a day in the animal foods he or she eats. Typically, a person will absorb about half of that, and the remainder will quickly pass from the intestine into the stool.

Different animal foods contain different levels of dietary cholesterol. Most lean meats contain around 80 mg of cholesterol per three-ounce serving and ten grams of fat. Caviar contains about 50 mg of cholesterol per tablespoon, three ounces of shrimp about 150 mg. Crab, lobster, and clams have half that amount of cholesterol and very little fat.

The food with the highest amount of cholesterol per serving, by the way, would probably be calf brains—2000 mg for a serving of three ounces. Calf brain consumption is so low that the net effect on the cholesterol intake of the general public is negligible.

How much cholesterol do eggs contain?

We note here that recent United States Department of Agriculture estimates have revised the cholesterol amounts present in a large egg. Previously, the amount of cholesterol present was estimated at 274 mg. As a result of advances in egg production technology and more sophisticated testing methods, the current figure is a little over 213 mg (a reduction of 22 percent). While eggs still contribute high levels of cholesterol to the American diet, the new information is likely to be good news for those who are limiting their cholesterol intake in consultation with a physician.

It also seems appropriate to comment here on a recent scientific development that has garnered quite a bit of attention. Food scientists have apparently developed techniques that can reduce the cholesterol content of milk by half. While commercial applications are still some years away, many in the low-cholesterol camp have hailed the announcement as a breakthrough.

For all practical purposes, though, the main difference the consumer is going to notice in these products, assuming they do eventually make it to market, is a higher price tag. The actual amounts of cholesterol in question are quite small.

Whole milk averages only about 35 mg of cholesterol per 8-ounce serving, with 9 grams of fat. Assuming that one drinks 3 such glasses a day, that is still just 115 mg of cholesterol and 27 grams of fat. Actually, most consumers would be ingesting even less, considering the popularity of low-fat and skim milk.

It is also worth noting that the National Cholesterol Education Program's "recommended" maximum level of intake of dietary cholesterol (300 mg/day) is arbitrary and more or less meaningless from a physiological standpoint. The figure does not represent any demonstrated change in risk in any clinical study.

Serum cholesterol

What does the term "serum cholesterol" mean?

Serum is the clear, liquid part of clotted blood that can be separated in the laboratory by centrifugation. Serum cholesterol, then, is the cholesterol that is present in the serum sample. Serum cholesterol levels are customarily reported in terms of milligrams per deciliter, or mg/dl. A milligram is 1/1000th of a gram, or about 1/30,000th of an ounce; a deciliter is 1/10th of a liter, or about 1/5 of a pint. The serum level of cholesterol varies between 140 and 300 mg/dl in healthy people.

Even at the extremely high serum cholesterol level of 300 mg/dl, the concentration of cholesterol in serum is, in physical terms, minute—about .03 percent of serum. Nonetheless, levels of serum cholesterol above 240 mg/dl are connected with a significantly increased risk of coronary heart disease (or CHD for short). This much is accepted within the scientific community. However, as will become clear in the following pages, there is considerable controversy concerning the assessment of the risks associated with lower serum cholesterol levels.

Dietary and serum cholesterol—the differences

What is the difference between dietary and serum cholesterol?

Dietary cholesterol is in all foods derived from animals. Daily intake levels of dietary cholesterol can vary from zero (among strict vegetarians) to 1,500 mg (among people who eat extremely large quantities of eggs).

Serum cholesterol, by contrast, is the concentration of cholesterol in our blood. Its high and low ends are much less extreme than the dietary intake levels.

More important, serum cholesterol levels in any individual can be totally unrelated to the amount of cholesterol consumed.

Most Americans have come to recognize serum cholesterol levels as a risk factor for CHD. What has received less attention, however, is the fact that blood cholesterol levels represent *one risk factor of many*—and that the degree to which any given citizen can benefit from dietary changes designed to lower serum cholesterol is a matter of heated debate in the scientific community.

Fats

What are fats?

Many health authorities believe that Americans are eating too much fat. The general trend in eating habits in the United States has been toward a diet that relies less on fatty foods. Nevertheless, there still are a number of questions surrounding the issue of fats in our diet that remain unclear for many people.

Fats are the oily or greasy substances in foods and animal tissues. They are insoluble in water but can be dissolved in substances like alcohol or ether.

The most familiar fats are probably the visible ones. These would include the fats in salad and cooking oils, butter, margarine, mayonnaise, bacon grease, and the external fat on meat. Visible fats make up nearly half of our usual fat intake.

The other half, typically, is obtained from hidden or "invisible" fats (in other words, fats not readily seen in foods). Included in this group would be the fats contained in such foods as nuts, lean meats, potato chips, candy, pastries, whole grains, and many others.

What are "invisible" fats?

The term "lipid" is sometimes used interchangeably with "fat"—but it's actually somewhat broader in meaning. Lipids include fats, oils, and other fatty substances extracted with alcohol, including cholesterol, pigments, fat-soluble vitamins, and complex fats that contain phosphorus or sugar.

Saturated fat

The term "saturated fat" is a familiar one to most Americans, but the underlying meaning is often not entirely clear. Saturation refers to the degree to which the carbons present in the fat react with hydrogen. If all the available bonds are occupied by hydrogen, the fat is considered saturated.

If two carbon bonds are not fully occupied with hydrogen and contain only one atom of hydrogen, so that they have one double bond, the term "monounsaturated" is used. If four carbon atoms are not fully occupied with hydrogen and contain only one hydrogen atom each, so that they have two double bonds, scientists use the term "polyunsaturated." Some polyunsaturated fats may contain as many as six double bonds.

How much fat do Americans eat?

Presently, Americans consume on average 37 percent of their total calories from fat. This means that 63 percent of our calorie intake comes from other sources, namely carbohydrate, protein, and alcohol.

Approximately 15 percent of our caloric intake comes from saturated fat. Another 15 percent comes from monounsaturated fat, and the rest of the calories from fat come from polyunsaturated fat.

Are saturated fats "bad for you"?

It's true that saturated fat can raise cholesterol levels in the blood of many persons—but it doesn't do this in every case, or for every individual.

Are polyunsaturated fats "good for you"?

Studies show that the maximum effect attributable to increased consumption of saturated fat is between 10 and 30 mg/dl—roughly 10 percent of the total cholesterol for a person with a serum level of 200 mg/dl. Increases in polyunsaturated fat intakes are associated with a similar, minimal decrease (again, about 10 percent) in the blood cholesterol levels of some persons.

The studies that bear out these effects, however, are just that—studies. We should remember that no one eats a diet composed entirely of saturated fat, and very few people eat the elevated levels associated with clinical tests.

What's more important than measurable short-term changes in a person's serum cholesterol level, however, is the long-term effect of consumption of saturated fat. It is with this issue that some of the most surprising (and least-publicized) research concerning fat and our diet arises.

Several long-term, cross-sectional studies in the United States have shown that people on high-fat diets have, as a group, the same serum cholesterol levels as those who are on low-fat diets! The same is true for persons on different cholesterol intakes.

Are fats essential?

Fat is essential for human life. It is necessary as a vehicle for the absorption of fat-soluble vitamins and as a source of essential fatty acids. Relative to the overall levels of consumption, fat provides more energy than either protein or carbohydrate. Excess carbohydrate, in fact, is actually converted to fat in the human body.

Far from acting as a poison, fat is an important part of a good diet. While it is possible to eat a healthy vegetarian diet that does not feature any animal fat, it is *not* possible to eat a healthy diet that excludes all fats, animal- or vegetable-based.

Coronary heart disease

In the next chapter: an in-depth look at coronary heart disease.

Chapter Six: Coronary Heart Disease

The nation's number one killer

What is coronary heart disease?

Heart disease is the leading cause of death in the United States. Coronary heart disease (CHD) accounts for two-thirds of all heart disease. Other types of heart disease, such as congenital problems, injury to heart muscles due to high blood pressure, infection, degeneration, rheumatic fever, and vascular disease, make up the other third.

How many people die of CHD yearly?

CHD afflicts approximately five million people in our country and causes 550,000 deaths per year.

Most CHD results from plugging of the coronary arteries, associated with degeneration and narrowing of these arteries. These events may lead to clots that block the arteries, preventing nourishment of the heart tissues beyond the block. This narrowing process of plaque buildup in the medium and large arteries of the body is known as atherogenesis. (The overall result is known as atherosclerosis.) Men are at higher risk than women for atherogenesis because plaques begin to form at puberty in males—and two decades later in females.

Certainly the most threatening part of CHD is failure of coronary circulation, resulting in a "heart attack." This is characterized by chest pain, weakness, sweating, and a drop in blood pressure. In addition, these attacks are usually accompanied by a chaotic, irregular pulse rhythm, which interrupts blood flow to portions of the heart muscle. This reduction in blood flow causes injury to heart cells, which can severely impair the work capacity of the heart. Sudden death occurs in about one-third of the cases.

Risk factors

What is risk factor?

In general, traits that predict the occurrence of any disease—including CHD—are called risk factors. A risk factor is a measure that is correlated with the chance that a given individual has of developing a disease.

Risk factors are not necessarily direct causes of the disease, nor does their presence guarantee that the disease will occur in a given individual. By the same token, a factor's absence does not indicate that the disease will not occur, because there are multiple causes for most long-term diseases that afflict American adults. Some people without any of the known risk factors still develop CHD.

What risk factors are associated with CHD?

Established risk factors for CHD include family history and related genetic factors, increasing age, being male, cigarette smoking, high blood pressure, high serum cholesterol levels, obesity, physical inactivity, and diabetes. (There may even be more we haven't learned enough about yet, such as severe stress.) We should note that while high levels of serum cholesterol are risk factors, simply having a high blood cholesterol reading is not as significant as was once thought. The reason for this has to do with high- and low-density lipoproteins—the so-called "good" and "bad" types of cholesterol. Later in the book we will examine each type in detail.

The probability of developing CHD increases with the number and severity of risk factors present in a given individual. The increase in risk is more rapid in the presence of many risk factors than it would be if each risk factor were calculated separately.

Risk factors you cannot control

Can all risk factors be modified?

Some risk factors, like age, sex, and heredity, are not modifiable. Together, these factors account for about 35 percent of the total risk—more than any single modifiable risk factor.

In other words, if you are male, you have a greater risk of CHD than a female, and there is nothing you can do to change this. In addition, the risk can be further augmented by increased age and genetic predisposition that may be present in your case and absent in the cases of others.

"Premature death"

Obviously, in discussing CHD we take as our main objective the reduction of premature death resulting from the disease. Most people would be surprised to learn that roughly 40 percent of coronary deaths occur in people over 80 years of age. It is difficult, if not impossible, to regard people in this category as victims of premature death.

How old are most victims of CHD?

Only 7 percent of the deaths from CHD occur before age 55. Between the ages of 55 and 65, the figure is about 15 percent. Thus, nearly 8 out of 10 deaths from CHD occur after age 65.

CHD, then, is primarily a disease that strikes older people, though this is not the impression most Americans have been left with over the past few years. The combined effect of most of the advertisements and health organization warnings that concern themselves with cholesterol (and, by inference, heart disease) has been to convey a markedly different image of the person at risk of this health problem.

The image is that of a man between 45 and 55 years of age. He is a busy executive and a concerned family man. He may have "too much stress" in his daily life. He is not particularly overweight, but he does eat foods "high in saturated fat and dietary cholesterol." He is, it is strongly suggested, the typical individual at risk of CHD.

What are the major unmodifiable risk factors?

The major factors missing in the above depiction concern two important elements we cannot change at all. In most discussions of CHD, we are rarely informed of the importance of age or genetic predisposition toward heart disease as risk indicators. Age may be the single most important nonbehavioral factor related to risk of CHD, and one's genetic background is probably almost as important. Unfortunately, we cannot choose whether or not to age, and we cannot choose the genetic advantages or disadvantages passed on to us by our parents.

Risk factors you can control

Important modifiable risk factors for CHD include cigarette smoking, high blood pressure, and high serum cholesterol levels (principally low-density lipoprotein cholesterol). Together, these account for 60 percent of our CHD risk. Another 5 percent of the known risk is related to obesity, diabetes, and physical inactivity. Unmodifiable factors, as mentioned, account for 35 percent of the risk associated with CHD.

While risk factors like obesity and smoking may be considered modifiable, since it is always (in theory) possible to stop smoking or lose weight, such problems are usually not solved overnight. Similarly, it is not an easy matter in every case to lower serum cholesterol levels for any meaningful period of time. (As we will learn later, it is often impossible!)

Cholesterol may make the headlines, but when it comes to CHD, cholesterol is really not the whole story. To get an idea of the total risk picture, we must take a brief look at the other major alterable risk factors for CHD.

Smoking

How important is smoking as a CHD risk factor?

We all know that cigarette smoking represents a major threat to overall good health. Cigarette smoking is also the single most significant modifiable risk factor for CHD.

If you smoke, you court not only diseases like lung cancer and emphysema but you also dramatically increase your risk of a heart attack. Now and then you may hear arguments from the cigarette companies that "further research" is necessary before conclusions can be drawn on this subject, but this is nothing more than a semantic dodge. The research has been in for many years now, and the conclusion is inescapable: cigarette companies make products that kill their customers. (The many antismoking efforts conducted over the years by the Surgeon General's office illustrate the seriousness of the problem.)[1]

Can smokers who quit return to the risk levels of non-smokers?

Fortunately, when it comes to heart disease, those smokers who do achieve the difficult goal of quitting can quickly regain the ground that has been lost. A person who once smoked heavily, but quits, will, after a few years, have the same statistical risk as a lifetime nonsmoker with regard to CHD.

After adjustments for age are taken into account, it is estimated that smoking, as a risk factor, represents 22 percent of the total risk of CHD. (Note: all the following figures related to percentage of risk of CHD are age-adjusted.)

High blood pressure

High blood pressure, or hypertension, is also a major risk factor for CHD. Some 20 to 25 percent of the American adult population has high blood pressure. More than half of these have hypertensive heart disease (that is, an observable effect upon the function of the heart, such as enlargement, weakness, or even cardiac failure).

How important is high blood pressure as a CHD risk factor?

The great majority of people with mild hypertension do not know they have the disease, and undergo no treatment program. This is unfortunate, because elevated blood pressure is an important public health problem, above and beyond its role as a risk factor for CHD. The disease is common, presents no early symptoms, and is often lethal if left untreated. The proper treatment of mild to moderate high blood pressure, however, can have striking positive effects: clinical trials have resulted in significant decreases in overall and CHD mortality.

It is estimated that 20 percent of the overall risk of a heart attack is due to high blood pressure.

Obesity, diabetes, and inactivity

How important are obesity, diabetes, and inactivity as risk factors?

While these three factors contribute only 5 percent to the risk of CHD, their status as health problems should not be underestimated. Serious overweight, for example, contributes in complex ways to other known risk factors for CHD. Serum cholesterol levels may be higher in obese individuals, and high blood pressure is also more common in this group than in the rest of the population.

Of course, it is consistent with general good health to reach and maintain a reasonable weight and exercise regularly. Adult-onset diabetes, associated with obesity, can often be prevented by maintaining a reasonable weight.

For a full discussion of the health risks associated with excess body weight, see the later chapter on obesity and overweight.

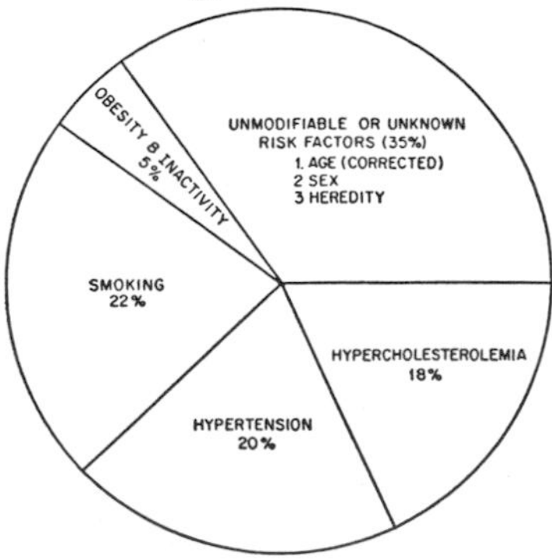

Figure 1. Risk for CHD attributable to specific factors (age-adjusted).

Serum cholesterol levels

High serum cholesterol levels do represent a risk factor for CHD; researchers estimate that this problem contributes about 18 percent of the total age-adjusted risk of the disease. However, most Americans have been presented with misleading information and unnecessarily alarming advice with regard to the following questions:

> *What constitutes a high serum cholesterol level?*
>
> *How does diet affect serum cholesterol levels?*
>
> *Can all people lower their serum cholesterol levels through dietary changes?*
>
> *Can dietary changes decrease every individual's risk of death from CHD?*

In the next chapter, we'll give the surprising answers to these questions—answers some of the most prominent health organizations in the country have ignored or glossed over.

Chapter Seven: Diet and Cholesterol Beyond the Scare

Eating scared

The way the foods we eat affect our risk of heart disease is a subject that has been wrenched out of context and profoundly exaggerated in recent years. Contrary to what many have come to believe, most Americans do not have significantly elevated serum cholesterol levels—and the few who do should be consulting a physician for advice, not advertisements, talk shows, or magazine articles.

Do most Americans have significantly elevated serum cholesterol levels?

The National Heart, Lung, and Blood Institute has developed a National Cholesterol Education

Program to increase awareness of the importance of serum cholesterol levels. Unfortunately, this group has been the source of as much exaggeration and misdirection as it has useful advice for physicians and their patients. The many examples of the Education Program's overzealous recommendations with regard to cholesterol will be examined in detail.

In addition, we will learn how the food you eat can affect your serum cholesterol level. We will look at how the terms used by many public health officials to categorize population groups have been slanted to cause unnecessary alarm about serum cholesterol. Finally, we will learn how the current consumption level of dietary cholesterol by Americans has been made to appear to be something it is not—namely, a serious public health problem.

Should I know my serum cholesterol level?

We preface all that follows with a word of advice: *learn your own serum cholesterol level and discuss your other possible risk factors with your physician.* Much of the current misinformation surrounding cholesterol and heart disease has been perpetuated through ill-advised attempts to diagnose and treat 250 million Americans for CHD at once. We make no such attempt here, and emphasize that nothing you read in this or any other book can take the place of a personal consultation with your doctor.

Regardless of your status with respect to other risk factors, you should know where you stand on blood cholesterol readings. Everyone over 20 should have his or her serum cholesterol levels measured on a regular basis and under conditions that assure accuracy—i.e., in the office of a physician who has access to a good laboratory.

The "good" cholesterol, "bad" cholesterol controversy

What are the so-called "good" and "bad" cholesterol types?

Although total serum cholesterol is a risk factor for CHD, newer knowledge has revealed that total serum cholesterol is not the most reliable indicator of risk. This is because total serum cholesterol includes a number of lipoproteins (that is, cholesterol bound to fats and proteins) that aid in the breakdown and transport of fat throughout the body. Two of these lipoprotein fractions alter risk associated with CHD—in opposite directions. These two lipoproteins (known as high- and low-density lipoproteins) are the much-discussed "good" and "bad" cholesterols. These media-coined terms, predictably, represent oversimplifications.

The point bears repeating: cholesterol itself is neither "good" nor "bad." The risk associated with cholesterol depends on how it is carried in the body.

The concentration of "bad" low-density lipoproteins (LDL) accelerates the buildup of plaque in the arteries and is an important risk factor. LDL is the most prominent lipoprotein found in human plasma and carries the most cholesterol (about 60 percent). "Good" high-density lipoproteins (HDL), on the other hand, are protective. As HDL levels rise, the risk of CHD is reduced.

Because of estrogenic hormones, women have a higher level of HDL and correspondingly lower levels of LDL until menopause. In contrast, men have a higher LDL/HDL ratio and, as a group, are at greater risk than women as far as CHD is concerned.

Do foods contain "good" or "bad" cholesterol?

As might be expected, the terms "good" and "bad" cholesterol have been the cause of much misunderstanding. Many people, upon being exposed to the first wave of headlines trumpeting the distinction, made the natural assumption that certain foods contained "good" or "bad" cholesterol. Obviously, this is impossible, since HDL and LDL are produced by the body itself.

The claim that LDL is the primary villain in the heart disease story, too, is a more black-and-white conclusion than the facts warrant. Atherosclerosis is a disease of multiple causes, in which the contribution to plaque buildup varies from individual to individual. In some cases, high levels of LDL may be important; in other cases, high LDL levels may be tolerated for years without clinical disease.

If your doctor does not provide you with information about your total cholesterol to HDL ratio, ask him or her to do so. It is possible that your total cholesterol value could be high but that your HDL level could indicate you are actually at very low risk! Remember, however, that the probability of developing CHD increases with the number of risk factors present in a given person—and with their severity.

Serum cholesterol and dietary cholesterol: which is the risk factor?

We saw in the previous chapter that serum cholesterol levels in any individual can be totally unrelated to the amount of cholesterol eaten. This is a crucial distinction that is usually ignored in discussions of cholesterol as a risk factor.

Is dietary cholesterol a risk factor?

Serum cholesterol (the cholesterol present in your blood) is a risk factor for CHD, whereas dietary cholesterol (the cholesterol present in food) is not.

Current research may be complex and occasionally contradictory, but one thing that is clear is that the current recommendation that adults consume no more than 300 mg/day of dietary cholesterol is not based on any consideration of how that level might affect someone's risk of heart disease. This recommendation, first proposed by the American Heart Association and later taken up by a number of other organizations including the National Cholesterol Education Program (NCEP), is completely arbitrary.

Furthermore, the difference between the American population's average level of consumption—perhaps 400 mg/day for an adult—and the current recommended maximum of 300 mg/day represents a trivial and probably irrelevant difference from a public health standpoint.

We note here that an expert committee in the United Kingdom in 1984 concluded that it could make no recommendation to the British public related to dietary cholesterol. The committee concluded that "the current intake of 350-450 mg/day is not excessive, and . . . evidence of [the effect of] this level of intake on blood cholesterol is inconclusive.'' This is the judgment passed on levels between 16 and 50 percent higher than the NCEP's recommended level!

How does what you eat affect your serum cholesterol level?

Sadly, the American recommended maximum intake guideline is not the only source of misleading advice with regard to dietary cholesterol. Sensational media coverage has led to numerous unfortunate misconceptions. There is a common notion, for instance, not only that dietary cholesterol is automatically linked to elevated blood cholesterol levels but that the cholesterol absorbed goes directly to one's heart, where it busily sets to work clogging up the arteries. Both ideas are simplistic and therefore popular with those who must write news copy. Both ideas, however, are wrong.

How important is diet in regulating serum cholesterol?

How important is dietary cholesterol in the control of serum cholesterol? Both dietary fat and dietary cholesterol play a role in determining the serum cholesterol level, but the response is highly variable from individual to individual. In short-term studies, dietary cholesterol has been shown to be less important in altering serum levels than saturated and polyunsaturated fats.

Dietary cholesterol does exert a minor upward effect on the serum cholesterol levels of some people, particularly if the diet is also high in saturated fat. That does not mean, however, that dietary fat and cholesterol "cause" CHD in and of themselves.

We must keep in mind that whether or not a given person consumes a great deal of dietary fat and cholesterol may be meaningless, since only about half of the adult population can affect serum cholesterol levels by altering the diet—and even then, the change is usually only on the order of 10 percent in either direction. The key is to identify where significant risk thresholds associated with serum cholesterol levels begin, rather than to establish dietary guidelines that are not scientifically sound.

Here is what we know. At dietary cholesterol consumption levels of 1500 mg/day (a mark, by the way, that's 500 percent of the "recommended" level!)—the serum cholesterol levels of *some*, but not all, test participants rise by an average of about 10 percent. Such elevated levels, however, do not suggest that imminent heart disease awaited the participants whose blood cholesterol levels rose. Serum cholesterol, we must remember, is a risk factor—not a sign of disease!

Furthermore, the important question about dietary intake is not how serum levels react in the short term but how the body itself adjusts over time to consumption of cholesterol. In most people, the body reacts by reducing its own synthesis (manufacture) of this essential substance.

Can the body adjust to varying levels of cholesterol intake?

This is what's missing in most discussions of the dietary fat and cholesterol issue—an appreciation that the human body itself acts as a small but exceedingly sophisticated chemical factory. If you are a physiologically normal individual, your body constantly monitors what comes in and alters its own production of cholesterol in order to keep body stores constant and guarantee essential functions. And even in those people who exhibit modest short-term serum cholesterol increases or decreases due to diet, there is a general tendency in most for the serum cholesterol—over a period of years—to return to genetically determined levels.

How do short-term and long-term effects of dietary cholesterol differ?

Four separate studies (most prominently the Framingham Heart Study, monitoring over 5,000 individuals) have been unable to show significant long-term differences in the serum cholesterol levels of people who've developed a long-term habit of eating no eggs a day compared with those who've typically eaten three eggs a day.[1] (For further information on this startling finding, see the pamphlet issued by William Kannel and Tavia Gordon through the Department of Health, Education, and Welfare, *The Framingham Diet Study: Diet and the Regulation of Serum Cholesterol.*) The same is true for saturated fat in the diet.

The key to understanding such issues may rest in the way we frame our questions. In the example above, for instance, the correct question may not be "Do eggs raise serum cholesterol levels?" but rather, "Can humans adapt, over a period of years, to diets that contain varying amounts of dietary cholesterol?"

As we've noted, it is true that short-term studies conducted over a period of six weeks or so can show an increase or decrease in serum cholesterol values of about 10 percent. Certain foods that can raise levels in these settings, whether eggs, foods containing saturated fats, butter, or any of the other current bugaboos, are then cast as the villains in the debate because they "raise serum cholesterol levels." But the key point, and the point that is somehow never raised, is this: people do not eat for six weeks and then stop. They eat throughout their lifetimes.

Does the "8-Week Cholesterol Cure" work?

The failure to address this fact is conspicuous in many, if not most, popular books and articles on the topic of cholesterol. Particularly troubling is the advice offered in the currently popular *8-Week Cholesterol Cure.* This regimen, predictably, takes advantage of the short-term changes that can occur through diet modifications, though the book's title clearly implies something more. What it implies is that after eight weeks of following the book's plan, no further diet or drug treatment is necessary for persons with significantly elevated cholesterol levels. This is patently false. (For more on the dubious claims of this regimen, see the section on "Dangerous Diets" beginning on page 207.)

The authors of this book believe that for most individuals the crucial question is not what happens in the short term but how the body reacts over a period of years. Indeed, there is growing evidence, including the studies on egg and fat consumption mentioned above, that the body can often adapt, over time, to whatever diet it receives.

This is not to suggest for a moment that there aren't certain individuals who can benefit from a medically supervised serum cholesterol reduction program in order to lower a significant risk of heart disease. There are indications, however, that those who are currently summoning the nation to attention with regard to this issue may be misreading the research and underestimating the corrective powers of the human body.

How important are the body's long-term adjustments to dietary cholesterol intake?

To put it another way, there are both short-term and long-term adjustments that the body makes to dietary change. By emphasizing only the short-term reactions and ignoring the long-term modifications the body makes to insure its own proper functioning, we cannot fully appreciate the role dietary fats and cholesterol actually play with regard to human health.

In fact, one of the long-term adjustments seems to be that *despite* their diets, people tend to develop diseases determined largely by genes (CHD, for example), and that family history, rather than any dietary pattern, plays a more dominant role in determining survival. (And by long-term, we mean over a lifetime—not the weeks or months monitored in most dietary studies.)

After age 55, serum cholesterol levels do not predict the risk of heart disease because of the growing importance of unmodifiable risk factors. This fact takes on tremendous significance when we realize that people over 55 are the group that should be most concerned about CHD!

How significant are serum cholesterol levels as predictors of heart disease for people over 55?

There is a great deal of compensation over the long term that the body makes—compensation that seems to steer individuals toward their genetic potential for serum cholesterol levels. In addition, the long-term studies that have been done on this subject indicate a tendency even for those with high serum cholesterol levels to creep back toward normal readings over eight, nine, ten or more years—regardless of their dietary patterns![2]

While we're discussing misconceptions associated with CHD and diet, here's another startling fact. In seven studies, incorporating over 47,000 participants for periods ranging from five to ten years, diet and drug intervention aimed at CHD had *no effect* on overall mortality.[3]

Do dietary and drug intervention aimed at CHD increase life span?

In layman's terms, this means that the test cases simply didn't live any longer than control groups as a result of intervention—even though the incidence of heart disease declined about 20 percent.

Now, this is certainly not offered in defense of the idea that all intervention against heart disease is useless. But it is worth knowing, for the sake of perspective, that many who adjust modifiable risk factors and don't die of heart disease, according to currently available information, don't gain any appreciable increase in life expectancy. Health problems other than CHD seem to negate any extension of the life span.

The doctor says my cholesterol level is "borderline high." What do I do?

"Borderline high"

The question of what constitutes an unacceptably high serum cholesterol level—and why—is an extremely controversial one in the scientific community. Yet that is not the impression most Americans receive from the media and many public health officials.

For most of us, the fact that a certain health recommendation receives substantial news coverage and is the subject of an expensive public awareness campaign is enough to convince us of the validity of that position. As we'll see, such trust is perhaps too easily placed.

The NCEP has advised that less than 200 mg/dl of total cholesterol and 130 mg/dl of LDL cholesterol are "desirable" for adults. Furthermore, they recommend that values between 200 and 239 mg/dl of total serum cholesterol, with 130-160 mg/dl of LDL cholesterol, should be considered "borderline high."

This is a contradiction in terms. Is such a serum cholesterol reading borderline, or is it high? In medicine, "borderline" means a grey zone between normal and diseased persons—a grey zone that usually requires no intervention.

On the other hand, if "borderline high" is really meant to suggest "high," then slightly less than half of the American adult population—that portion with blood cholesterol levels above 200 mg/dl—has dangerously elevated serum cholesterol levels and is in need of intervention. If this is what the NCEP is claiming, where is the evidence?

Are "undesirable" cholesterol levels "dangerous" ones?

Certainly, if the NCEP implies that readings over 200 mg/dl are "undesirable," that is not the same as claiming such levels are "dangerous." Nevertheless, considering the authority such pronouncements command, the message most Americans receive is likely to be one that connects grave health risks with the "borderline high" category.

Are such ideas accurate? Is, for instance, a 3- to 4-percent increase in total attributable risk of CHD (from a serum cholesterol reading of 230 mg/dl) really dangerous from a statistical standpoint, warranting immediate dietary changes regardless of whether other risk factors are present? This is the clear implication of the NCEP, but the available medical statistics do not support such a conclusion.

What constitutes an "undesirable" serum cholesterol level?

Furthermore, declaring that blood cholesterol levels over 200 mg/dl do not fall into the "desirable" category begs the question of whose "desires" are being taken into account. Not those of the countless reputable scientists and practitioners who consider a blood cholesterol reading in the NCEP's "borderline high" range to be quite normal.

In today's media-sensitive environment, wouldn't it make sense to ask that the medical advice being rendered by organizations such as the NCEP deal with incontrovertible, demonstrated, and significant health risks? If there are "grey areas" involved, wouldn't common sense and simple professionalism demand that this fact be acknowledged openly to patients and public alike?

Such concerns were apparently considered irrelevant (or not considered at all) by the NCEP. Nevertheless, their ominous-sounding "borderline high" distinction would probably be taken by most citizens to represent the most important risk threshold on the scale—the mark at which a dangerously elevated risk of CHD first surfaces. This is not the case.

What serum cholesterol readings reflect a significant risk?

For most adult Americans, the most significant benchmark is a serum cholesterol reading at or in excess of 240 mg/dl, LDL cholesterol in excess of 160 mg/dl, and a ratio of total cholesterol to HDL cholesterol of 4.0 or higher. This is the next step up from the NCEP's "borderline high."

Why is this level significant? It is at 240 mg/dl that the risk of CHD doubles, compared with a baseline of 200 mg/dl. At higher levels, the risk continues to rise sharply; above 300 mg/dl, the risk is 5 times greater.*

*For reasons of simplicity and ease of comparison, we will refer in subsequent pages to the 240 mg/dl level as describing the entrance into the "high-risk" group. However, as has been noted, what is critical in the determination of your risk is the ratio of total cholesterol to HDL cholesterol. Your serum cholesterol reading is essentially incomplete without this measurement, and your doctor should supply it when you have your blood cholesterol level checked. A ratio of 4.0 or higher connotes significantly increased risk.

In most cases, at 240 mg/dl, with a total cholesterol to HDL ratio of 4.0 or higher, you should be seeing a physician regularly and working out a comprehensive plan for lowering your blood cholesterol levels. Such efforts are particularly important for those with additional risk factors such as smoking, high blood pressure, obesity, being male, and/or having a family history of CHD. (As we've noted earlier, the higher your serum cholesterol, the more you should be concerned about other risk factors.)

Eighty-four percent of all Americans over 15 years of age have total serum cholesterol values below 240 mg/dl. (In addition, virtually *every* child under 15 would have a lower cholesterol level.)

There are risks . . . and there are risks

Some proponents of extremely conservative approaches to this issue buttress their arguments by citing "increased risk" at various levels below 240 mg/dl in epidemiological studies. The simple fact that statistical risk increases as blood cholesterol levels get higher is a truism; little or no meaningful information is gained by setting the lowest possible threshold.

The critical objective is to find the point at which a risk ceases to be a *reasonable* risk, and in our view that point is clearly 240 mg/dl. Risk, of course, is incurred by the very act of getting out of bed in the morning and going to work, but it does not therefore follow that the entire American workforce should stay in bed 24 hours a day.

Disputed ground

What underlies the dispute about "high" serum cholesterol levels?

There is, we must remember, considerable disagreement on the issue of exactly when a physician should tell a patient that his or her cholesterol level is "too high." For one thing, consensus conferences on CHD often do not adequately reflect the opinions of the nation's physicians. For another, determining the riskiest serum cholesterol levels is an issue on which many reasonable authorities in the health field simply disagree. Public health officials should recognize this difference of opinion for what it is—not paper it over.

Shifting standards

A few years ago, serum cholesterol levels were considered to be abnormally high when they reached 275 mg/dl in a middle-aged male. This was because such a reading placed the person in the 95th percentile—the top 5 percent, or "high end"—of the population group.

Similar methods were employed for other groups. This approach, then, identifies approximately 5 percent of the United States population as carrying an extremely high risk of CHD—a risk that should be modified through diet or drugs, under the supervision of a physician.

For many experienced medical professionals, that method was not sufficient. And an argument can be made that more than 5 percent of the American public should be engaged in efforts to lower blood cholesterol levels. The methods for determining what that segment is, however, should be sounder than what has thus far been put forward.

Change for change's sake

There is no demonstrated benefit associated with diet modifications designed to reduce serum cholesterol for people whose serum cholesterol levels fall below 240 mg/dl. Dr. William Taylor of the Beth Israel Hospital in Boston has calculated in his paper *Cholesterol Reduction and Life Expectancy:*

A Model Incorporating Multiple Risk Factors that *life-long* dietary intervention to reduce serum cholesterol levels in this group (which few can be expected to undergo) could be expected to extend life expectancy by only a few days.[4]

The Minnesota Coronary Survey tracked 9,057 adults between 30 and 70 years of age over more than 4 years. Half of the participants were given a diet low in saturated fat and cholesterol but high in polyunsaturated fat. The other half ate what most of us would consider a standard diet. There was a lowering of the average serum cholesterol level in the treated group, *but there was no decrease in the incidence of CHD.* The research is quite clear on the question; people in the 200-239 mg/dl "borderline high" group do not benefit over time from dietary changes that are aimed at lowering serum cholesterol levels.

Do people in the "borderline high" group benefit from dietary changes?

You *can* say that, as a general rule, these people should eat a balanced diet and watch their consumption of total calories, including those from saturated fats—but that's essentially true for all American adults!

Those behind the cholesterol scare would have the general public believe something that they cannot come out and say. They would have us believe that for people with cholesterol levels between 200 and 239 mg/dl, there is a clinically demonstrated decrease in mortality from CHD, a decrease that is attributable to dietary changes. This is simply not so.

Even though it is possible to observe short-term changes in serum cholesterol rates in some people through dietary change, it is *not* possible to track any statistically significant decrease in the rate of CHD to the so-called "borderline high" group. Apparently that fact is one the American Heart Association, the American Medical Association, the National Institutes of Health, the National Cholesterol Education Program, and the National Academy of Sciences prefer to ignore.

Chapter Eight: Why the Cholesterol Hype Is Hazardous

Science or semantics?

We've noted that by beginning at 200 mg/dl, the "borderline high" and "high" levels, when combined, describe a group consisting of nearly half of all American adults. It is tempting to conclude that many of those who established and promoted the current guidelines were driven, at least in part, by a desire to conduct a major, well-budgeted public health campaign and to reach the greatest possible number of people regardless of their status as risk group members.

One can almost envision the argument in committee rooms and department meetings across the country: "We need this money to save lives. Look—half of the country falls into the undesirable category!"

The public health profession's efforts would be more laudable had they targeted and identified those at legitimately high risks for CHD due to elevated LDL cholesterol levels. That other motives than this have come into play seems to us both likely and unfortunate.

"High risk"

What is the "high-risk strategy"?

We have reached perhaps the most important question in the cholesterol debate—and one that has not yet been adequately discussed. It is the question of whether CHD is still a problem to be addressed primarily by physicians, one-on-one with their patients, or a health issue that should be addressed through education of the whole population.

All acknowledge that the people who are in greatest need of preventive medical care for serum cholesterol problems are the 16 percent who fall into the legitimate "high-risk" category above 240 mg/dl.

These are the people whose genetic and metabolic tendencies have somehow worked against them. They present specific problems for physicians that demand individual diagnosis and careful treatment, not posters, slogans, and ad campaigns. Approaching this high-risk group through screening by a physician for the presence of risk factors and through follow-up treatment is a sound, proven approach known as the "high-risk strategy."

Intervening on a mass scale with people who are more or less normal with regard to the risk of CHD is unnecessary, often counterproductive with regard to reaching high-risk persons, and, perhaps most important, a waste of money.

Yet, the American Heart Association, the National Heart, Lung, and Blood Institute (through the NCEP), and the National Academy of Sciences (through its report on "Diet and Health") have all urged all Americans *from age two upward* to go on restricted diets in the hope of preventing CHD.

The idea of suggesting that a child of two years of age be placed on a low-fat, low-cholesterol diet in order to reduce the risk of CHD 50 years later is incomprehensible. The plugging of arteries associated with CHD does not even *begin* in males until middle adolescence, and two decades later than that in females. How on earth can small children benefit from such a diet? How, indeed, can the 84 percent of American adults whose serum cholesterol levels are not in the "high" category benefit from following these instructions?

Children and cholesterol

What about children and cholesterol?

On the emotional subject of children and cholesterol, we quote the Committee on Nutrition of the American Academy of Pediatrics.

"[T]he Committee . . . does not favor universal testing of blood cholesterol levels of children either in the hospital or in the office of the private physician [for a number of reasons] . . . [T]he measurement of cholesterol is fraught with difficulties . . . [and] a single blood cholesterol level in children [or adults] may not reflect day-to-day and seasonal variations. [In addition,] a sporadic elevated concentration of cholesterol in a child with no high-risk family history of coronary heart disease could lead to the initiation of severe dietary control that would be difficult to maintain in a growing child. In fact, such an unwarranted diet or treatment could be deleterious to growth and development."[1]

Established benefits

Public health measures should have established benefits. If a measure has no benefit, it should not be instituted. These are basic principles supposedly familiar to anyone with a background in public health, but one can't help wondering if perhaps they have been forgotten in the last few years.

High serum cholesterol, it bears repeating, is *not a disease* and is not synonymous with CHD. Furthermore, contrary to what the general public has been led to believe, nothing resembling a meaningful consensus has, as yet, developed on important issues related to serum cholesterol as a risk factor for heart disease—issues such as nationwide dietary guidelines and the "borderline high" controversy. By implying that such a consensus does exist, public health officials, the media, and the food industry have exaggerated and perpetuated a "health crisis" that centers on uninformed overreaction to cholesterol's role as a risk factor for CHD.

That charge may sound harsh at first, but not when one realizes that the battle against CHD waged over the past two decades *is being won, not lost!* This fact is virtually unknown to the American public, which receives just the opposite impression from those who should certainly know better.

Progress in meeting the challenge of heart disease

Is death due to CHD increasing?

The rate of CHD is declining in this country at a pace of 2 percent per year. This adds up to roughly 40 percent since 1968, a remarkable abatement of CHD frequency.

This drop in CHD mortality, largely of unknown cause, began before there was any significant education effort about risk factors, including cholesterol levels. Based on the information we receive about our diets, however, most of us would probably guess that CHD mortality had increased in recent years, primarily because of the foods we eat. That this widespread misunderstanding should be skillfully exploited, rather than corrected, is troubling in the extreme. Americans deserve better and more complete information than they have received on this subject. It is clear enough to us that the National Cholesterol Education Program is not the organization to provide this information.

When to sound the alarm

By way of comparison, it seems fair to note that the all-encompassing, no-holds-barred, get-the-message-out-loud-and-clear media campaign does indeed have its place in the public health arena. The many efforts to counteract smoking, drug addiction, or the practices linked to the AIDS epidemic, for example, were and are highly praiseworthy. Consumption of generous amounts of saturated fat and cholesterol, as a health risk, is simply not in the same league.

Smoking kills people. If you smoke, you confront perhaps the single most significant behaviorally rooted threat to your health. You endanger the health of others around you with second-hand smoke. You dramatically increase your chances of dying from lung cancer, emphysema, or heart disease. If you quit smoking, on the other hand, you can regain much of the ground you lost during the time you smoked. It is excellent public health policy to mount high-visibility campaigns that alert people to the dangers of smoking and offer suggestions as to how they can quit.

Consuming saturated fat and dietary cholesterol, in stark contrast, is by no means the most important

CHD risk factor; it is related remotely, in some individuals, to CHD. Severely restricting your dietary fat and cholesterol intake may not affect your blood cholesterol level in the slightest, because millions of Americans cannot change these levels through dietary means. Lower blood cholesterol levels may not have any significant effect on your overall life expectancy. What's more, your serum cholesterol level may not even be the most important factor in your overall risk of CHD. In fact, very low serum cholesterol levels—those below 160 mg/dl—are associated with increased mortality in persons of middle age and older.

Edinburgh University's Professor Michael Oliver, a distinguished researcher in this area, argues that increases in serum cholesterol levels that take place as we age might be part of an adaptation process necessary to maintain the health of cell membranes. If this is true, Professor Oliver's observation can serve as the final refutation of the simplistic but widely accepted view that low cholesterol levels are always synonymous with desirable cholesterol levels.[2]

Cholesterol—compared with smoking

Is lowering serum cholesterol levels as important as quitting smoking?

People tend to equate the current campaign to lower dietary cholesterol intake with the anti-smoking efforts begun in the early Sixties. The two cases are not comparable.

In a perfect world, we would ask heavy smokers who are also fond of eating extremely large amounts of eggs and fatty meats to stop smoking and adopt a more sensible diet. If forced to choose only one lifestyle change, however, such people are significantly better off trying to stop smoking, and continuing their present diets, than going about things in the opposite order.

Smoking is a health hazard as serious and well documented as any we face. Dietary fat and cholesterol are so insignificant when compared with the health risks associated with smoking that it is simply inappropriate to equate the two.

No "chicken soup" public health policies, please

How sound are our public health priorities?

As most Americans are aware, a great deal of time and effort has been expended in recent years urging people to modify their diets in an effort to reduce serum cholesterol levels. It should be clear now, though, that for most of us the risks are not as clear-cut as we have been led to believe.

For many, however, there is the tendency to offer the "chicken soup argument." "It can't hurt," some maintain, "and it might even help—so why not?"

There are a number of excellent reasons why not. To begin with, we repeat the fundamental principle that all public health initiatives should have a proven benefit. Attempts to reduce dietary fat and cholesterol intake on a mass scale do not meet this standard.

Significantly elevated blood cholesterol levels are a problem for only a fraction of American adults. Healthy premenopausal women and preteen children are virtually immune to CHD. Why should we ask these groups to alter their diets dramatically?

To the extent that there is a problem with elevated serum cholesterol levels in this country, the problem affects specific people who must be evaluated by qualified physicians on a case-by-case basis. Trumpeting the "good word" to the entire population (most of whom have nothing to worry about) dilutes the message and may even devalue it.

Also worth taking into account is the simple pointlessness of unnecessary alarm. Most Americans have quite enough to worry about these days and shouldn't be asked, for no good reason, to fret over one of life's remaining genuine pleasures—eating.

Actually, the fact that there are so many other things to worry about—legitimate things—leads us to the final, crucial reason why the cholesterol scare is bad for America. *There are simply too many other serious problems to which we could be committing the resources.*

"Why," we are often asked, "must you make such a fuss over the cholesterol issue?" In the troubled era in which we live, have we no better goals for our public health organizations? Can the energies and attention spans of most Americans be put to no better purpose than to worry over questions that are completely irrelevant to so many of them? Is the federal health budget spilling over with excess cash? Have other public health problems of much greater gravity, such as low birth weight among minority infants, the commercially lucrative perpetuation of nicotine addiction, and the AIDS virus, finally been solved?

With so many more pressing national health dilemmas, why must we so thoroughly confuse our priorities?

SECTION THREE: WHAT DO WE EAT?

Chapter Nine: Obesity and Overweight

Weighty issues

It should come as no surprise that millions of Americans weigh more than they should.

What health risks do these people face? How serious are they? What are the best and safest ways for people to lose weight? Are any diets actually dangerous?

Far too often, overweight Americans are the target of marketing efforts that do not provide anything resembling authoritative, helpful advice on weight loss. This section of the book will, we hope, help to supply some much-needed perspective.

Supermarket — or health spa?

The variety of pills, wafers, and powders available in your supermarket or drugstore to help in weight loss efforts can be bewildering. These products are only the most prominent evidence of a growing, thriving industry offering the promise of weight loss.

To the degree that this trend reflects a concern for watching one's total calorie consumption, the diet craze can be considered a positive development. Certainly overweight and the health risks that may accompany it are the most serious nutritional problems in the United States.

How helpful are commercial weight loss aids?

Many people today are very conscious of their weight, both for appearance's sake, and perhaps secondarily for health reasons. There is, accordingly, a large market for weight-loss products. Consumers must be careful, however, in selecting these products; few of them represent sound ways to achieve lasting weight reduction. The unfortunate fact is that with many of the commercially available weight-loss products too much emphasis has been placed on quick weight loss and not enough on long-term dietary goals.

The only effective means of losing weight is a reduction of caloric intake, combined with an exercise program that burns excess calories. (Elsewhere in this book, you'll find some suggested dietary guidelines that can help you attain your weight-loss goals.)

Many people look for ways around the difficult, long-term job of altering eating and exercise habits, and many companies are more than happy to provide "easy" diet programs that "work fast." Almost always, however, whatever weight is lost is regained just as quickly.

The reality for the vast majority of us is that for long-term maintenance of a reasonable weight, we must learn to live *with* food, not without it.

Reaching a reasonable weight and maintaining it is often very difficult. Most of the commercially available diet preparations won't change that in the slightest. It's worth remembering, too, that as you get older and you need fewer calories for actual sustenance, food can become a comfort and solace as much as a physical necessity. At the same time, exercise usually becomes more difficult as the years go by. Thus, weight maintenance can become quite a challenge as we age.

WHAT IS A CALORIE?

A calorie is a unit of measurement of energy. Technically, it is the amount of heat energy required to raise the temperature of one gram of water by one degree centigrade. It is a term commonly used in physics. For foods and the energy they provide, we use the term kilocalories, a value one thousand times that of a calorie. Thus, one kilocalorie is the amount of heat energy required to raise 1,000 grams of water (about a quart) one degree centigrade.

Kilocalorie, though, is a rather cumbersome term, so in recent years the kilocalorie was identified by using the term "Calorie" (that is, calorie spelled with a capital "c"). Currently, the word calorie, with a small "c," is generally used by nutritionists, the food industry, and physicians to express the caloric values of foods and of energy expenditures. This is the usage in this book as well.

An 8-ounce glass of whole milk, for instance, provides 160 calories; the same amount of skim milk provides 90 calories. For purposes of comparison, consider that a 140-pound individual walking briskly for 15 minutes expends 75 calories.

Calories are not nutrients. They are units of energy our body cells obtain from burning (or "metabolizing") the fat, carbohydrate, protein, and alcohol that we consume from foods and beverages.

Vitamins, minerals, and water do not provide calories, but they are necessary nutrients the body uses to metabolize the constituents of foods and beverages that supply us with energy and build body tissues.

Foods are described in terms of their total calories because that is the way we evaluate their energy content. Thus, fat provides approximately 9 calories per gram while carbohydrate (i.e., sugars and starches) and protein provide 4 calories per gram. Alcohol is in between, providing 7 calories per gram. Thus, if in a 24 hour period, one consumes 70 grams of protein, 100 grams of fat, 300 grams of carbohydrate, and 30 grams of alcohol, one's total consumption would be approximately 2,590 calories. ($370 \times 4 + 100 \times 9 + 30 \times 7 = 2{,}590$.)

Contrary to popular belief, there is really no such thing as an "empty calorie," just as there is no such thing as a "small gallon" of gasoline. All calories are full calories—full of energy! "Empty calories" is a misleading term commonly used to describe calories derived from a food or beverage that provides few or no valuable nutrients such as protein, vitamins, or minerals. When such foods or beverages (alcohol, for instance) are burned by the body, they provide only calories—though the calories still represent a specific amount of energy for the body.

On the other hand, when calories are obtained from fruit juices, milk, potatoes, or other foods, the nutrients in these foods are also consumed. In both categories, however, the calories are all equally "full" from an energy standpoint.

Animal vs. vegetable fats

Are animal fats more likely to make you overweight than other fats?

There is a widespread belief that animal fats provide more calories than vegetable-based ones. This is not so.

Fats and oils as they occur in foods or are added to foods all have the same number of calories—9 per gram, or about 270 per ounce. Thus, a pat of butter, usually figured at 5 grams, provides 45 calories, the same as a pat of margarine. A cup of corn oil has the same number of calories as a cup of any other kind of edible oil, i.e., 220 calories. And an ounce of meat fat has the same number of calories as an ounce of chicken fat or any other kind of fat.

Ounce for ounce, edible fats and oils all have the same caloric content.

Saturated fat

The difference between saturated fat and other types of dietary fat is a chemical one, not a caloric one. As we've noted, all fats, saturated, monounsaturated, or polyunsaturated, provide the same number of calories.

The fats in meats and whole milk products—milk, ice cream, and cheese—are the major sources of saturated fats in our diets. The so-called tropical oils, palm and coconut, vary in saturation from 49 to 80 percent. These tropical oils make up a very small amount of our total fat, however: only 1 to 2 percent, much less than meat and dairy fats, and hence are not important sources of fat in our diets.

What types of foods are high in saturated fats?

What kinds of foods are low in saturated fats?

Generally, vegetable fats such as soy, corn, olive, cottonseed, safflower, and canola, are low in saturated fats and therefore high in both mono- and polyunsaturated fats.

Because saturated fat has the same number of calories as unsaturated fat, it has the same potential to cause a weight problem. In present day American diets, fats provide 35 to 40 percent of total calories, with saturated fats providing 16 to 18 percent. Monounsaturated fats provide a similar amount, and polyunsaturated fats provide four to five percent.

Saturated fat has often been cast as the villain in the continuing debate over serum cholesterol levels. Some consider the use in the commercial food industry of tropical oils (which contain saturated fat) to be the equivalent of "poisoning" the

American public. The claim is unsupported by existing evidence. Consumption of tropical oils, on the whole, is a relatively insignificant factor in the American diet, and is certainly not the most important target in the ongoing efforts to reduce the amount of fat we eat.

What is hydrogenation?

I note that some fats are hydrogenated. What does this mean?

Hydrogenation is a chemical process by which hydrogen atoms are added to fat. The process does not increase the calories that the fat provides. It is done primarily to make a liquid oil into a solid or semisolid fat (such as a shortening). Hydrogenation also prolongs the shelf life of the oil, decreases the amount of monounsaturated and polyunsaturated fat, and increases the amount of saturated fat. Hydrogenated fats tend to raise serum cholesterol in some individuals more than vegetable oils. Hydrogenation is a controllable process.

Alcohol and calories

How can alcohol contribute to weight problems?

Alcohol is a potent source of calories—7 calories per gram, which is about twice as much as protein or carbohydrate and a little less than the same amount of fat.

The alcohol content of hard liquor is usually given in relation to its "proof," which is twice the percentage of alcohol. Thus, a whiskey or gin of 80 proof is 40 percent alcohol. The amount of alcohol in wine and beer is usually stated in percent by volume, with wines averaging around 12 percent and beer averaging 4 to 6 percent.

Obviously, for someone limiting calorie consumption, intake of large amounts of alcohol isn't a good idea. A more important reason not to drink excessively has to do with the many health and safety risks associated with alcohol abuse, not the least of which are motor vehicle accidents. Regardless of whether or not you are trying to lose weight, the Surgeon General suggests that, if you drink, you do so in moderation.

Who's obese?

Obesity usually describes someone who is 20 percent or more above his or her desirable weight due to an increase in body fat. When one is 40 percent or more above, the term morbid obesity is used. Researchers of recent years have devised more accurate definitions of obesity based on a comparison of body tissues—fat versus lean body mass. But this definition is too cumbersome for general use.

Some people, of course, are slightly over their desirable weights but could not be considered obese. 10 to 20 percent above the Metropolitan standards for your height and sex is considered overweight, rather than obese.

For some, of course, the mere fact of being overweight doesn't carry a great deal of significance. Athletes and others with highly developed muscle structures can be overweight, but not overfat. This is because frequent, strenuous muscular activity (exercise or hard physical work) enlarges the muscles used—and muscle has more protein and less fat than most other body tissues. Most of us, however, don't fall into this category.

Can you be overweight, but not overfat?

Defining obesity by a percentage above desirable weight brings us to the issue of what, exactly, someone's desirable weight is.

How can I determine my desirable weight?

In 1942, the Metropolitan Life Insurance Company studied thousands of records to determine at what weight, for specific heights, men and women lived the longest. These turned out, interestingly enough, to be the average weights for any height of each sex at age 30.

These weights were subsequently termed "ideal weights." The company decided (somewhat arbitrarily) to gauge the weights against three body frame sizes—small, medium, and large. In 1959, as a result of another study of more than 4 million insured people, the company announced new tables and referred to them as "Desirable Weight Tables." These figures turned out to be the average weight for a person of any given height and sex at age 25 and were slightly lower than the weights published in 1942.

The most recent weight distributions were published in 1983, also by the Metropolitan. For some heights and frame sizes, the standards are slightly higher than previous ones. This edition does not use the term "desirable"; instead, the company opted for the more objective title, "1983 Metropolitan Height and Weight Tables." However, the term "desirable" is still used by most physicians, nutritionists, and the public.

Thus, to find your desirable weight, simply use the following table. The Metropolitan standards are also available in many texts on nutrition, medicine, or health. Most physicians, nutritionists, and dietitians also have a copy of them. There is a range of a few pounds of weight in either direction for each height classification.

1983 Metropolitan Height and Weight Tables

Men

Height		*Small Frame*	*Medium Frame*	*Large Frame*
Feet	*Inches*			
5	2	128-134	131-141	138-150
5	3	130-136	133-143	140-153
5	4	132-138	135-145	142-156
5	5	134-140	137-148	144-160
5	6	136-142	139-151	146-164
5	7	138-145	142-154	149-168
5	8	140-148	145-157	152-172
5	9	142-151	148-160	155-176
5	10	144-154	151-163	158-180
5	11	146-157	154-166	161-184
6	0	149-160	157-170	164-188
6	1	152-164	160-174	168-192
6	2	155-168	164-178	172-197
6	3	158-172	167-182	176-202
6	4	162-176	171-187	181-207

Women

Height		*Small Frame*	*Medium Frame*	*Large Frame*
Feet	*Inches*			
4	10	102-111	109-121	118-131
4	11	103-113	111-123	120-134
5	0	104-115	113-126	122-137
5	1	106-118	115-129	125-140
5	2	108-121	118-132	128-143
5	3	111-124	121-135	131-147
5	4	114-127	124-138	134-151
5	5	117-130	127-141	137-155
5	6	120-133	130-144	140-159
5	7	123-136	133-147	143-163
5	8	126-139	136-150	146-167
5	9	129-142	139-153	149-170
5	10	132-145	142-156	152-173
5	11	135-148	145-159	155-176
6	0	138-151	148-162	158-179

Reprinted with permission from *Living Nutrition*, fourth edition, Fredrick J. Stare and Margaret McWilliams. Published by John Wiley & Sons.

Many health professionals (including the authors) much prefer the term "reasonable weight" to "desirable weight."

The Surgeon General's report *Nutrition and Health,* published in 1988, gives a figure of 34 million obese adults ages 20-74 years in the United States, with the highest obesity rate observed among the poor and minority groups. Estimates of the total number of overweight (but not obese) adults vary from 50 to 100 million. If we take the mean number of 75 million and add to it the mean number of those who are obese (34 million), we get an extremely rough but very troubling figure of 109 million adults who are either overweight or obese.

How many Americans are obese or overweight?

In our society, black women over 40 to 45 years of age are more likely to be obese than other groups. The reasons underlying this are complicated and still somewhat open to conjecture.

No reliable figures are available for the obesity rate among children or adolescents.

It's worth noting that Americans, as a group, are no more overweight or obese than citizens of other developed nations, with the significant exception of Japan.

Calories in, calories out

What is the cause of obesity?

There is really only one practical cause of obesity: the consumption of more total calories over a period of time than the calories expended. For an average adult, simple existence requires about 1,100-1,200 calories per day. These calories are needed to keep our bodies breathing, our hearts pumping, and to maintain a normal temperature (98.6 degrees Fahrenheit). (The calories are also required for certain muscular activities that take place even at rest.) This level of calorie consumption is called the Basal Metabolic Rate (BMR).

So much for the nutritional needs of someone who spends all day sitting passively, staring at the walls. For those of us who prefer to stand, walk, run, clean house, play tennis, swim, go to work, or do anything else, the body requires more calories—1,000 to 2,000 or more per day, depending upon the level of activity.

Thus, if your total daily caloric expenditure averages 2,500, and you consume an average of 2,500 calories from food and beverages, your weight will remain constant. But if you consume 2,500 calories per day and use only 2,000, you will gain weight—about one pound a week.

The reverse is also true. If you consume only 2,000 calories and use up 2,500, you will lose approximately one pound in a week. The body requires approximately 3,500 excess calories to gain a pound—and 3,500 calories under the amount used to lose a pound.

The cause of excess body weight, therefore, is really nothing complicated. It's simply a matter of consuming more calories than are expended over a given period of time.

Children and obesity

How serious a problem is obesity among children?

When the question of obesity among children arises, emotion often gets the better of the few facts available. We do not know of any data obtained from clinical studies involving large numbers of children. Our guess is that 25 to 30 percent of children are either overweight or obese, but fortunately most of them "grow out of it" during adolescence, so that by young adulthood few have kept their childhood obesity.

Most overweight or obese children are unlikely to benefit from a strict dietary program. Vigorous exercise, however, is another matter.

A sensible exercise program for children and adolescents is advisable, in part because such a program helps in forming habits that may carry over to adulthood. And certainly, there's no reason to limit these activities only to those children who have excess body weight.

Many studies have shown that most obese children and adolescents do not consume extremely large amounts of calorie-laden foods, but they are relatively inactive. Exercise is important in weight control at all ages and may be particularly helpful early on in life.

What are the dangers of restricting food intake among children?

We should note, in addition, that it can be extremely dangerous to place children on severe low-calorie and/or low-fat diets. (In the case of infants, restricting fat intake can result in death!) Children need adequate calories and varied diets selected from the Basic Four Food Groups to supply them with the 50 or more nutrients required for growth. Thus, austere restrictions of foods, no matter how well intentioned, can interfere with the proper development of their bodies.

Cholesterol and obesity

Broadly speaking, cholesterol intake from foods has nothing to do with obesity. Egg yolk is the only common food rich in cholesterol, yet a single egg yolk averages only 60 calories. Therefore, eating three yolks a day amounts to less than 200 calories.

What's the best way for obese people to try to lower serum cholesterol levels?

On the other hand, serum cholesterol is usually increased by obesity—more so than by the cholesterol content of the diet. The blood cholesterol level tends to decrease with loss of weight. In fact, for overweight and obese people, the loss of five to ten pounds can result in a reduction in the serum cholesterol levels—though for many, this drop will be a relatively short-term one. (Weight loss is also an effective way to lower your blood pressure.)

This will probably come as a surprise to those who follow complicated diets constituted expressly for the reduction of serum cholesterol levels. Nevertheless, such are the facts: for those of us with excess body weight, the simplest and best way to lower blood cholesterol levels—at least in the short term—is not to eat any one specific food in abundance—but simply to eat less of everything! Above and beyond this, of course, is the fact that maintaining a reasonable weight is associated with better health and longer life than being overweight.

What if I'm "genetically" overweight?

"Genetic" obesity

For those who come from families that experience more than their share of obesity and overweight, there are many puzzling questions.

Some wonder, for instance, whether it's true that there are certain people for whom obesity is a "normal" state—or at least highly likely from a genetic standpoint. If so, are health risks the same for such individuals? And what options are open to them to limit the health risks associated with obesity?

It has long been thought that some obesity is genetically based, but firm evidence to support this belief has been obtained only recently.

Nevertheless, all obesity is rooted in caloric imbalance, and the health risks associated with obesity are the same regardless of the cause. The only option that successfully limits the health risks of obesity over the long term, and for the rest of one's life, is to bring caloric intake (i.e., the foods you eat and the beverages you drink) into balance with caloric expenditure (i.e., physical activity and exercise). This represents the soundest approach for reaching and maintaining a reasonable weight.

How much can diet and exercise compensate for "genetic obesity"?

Diet and exercise can completely compensate for any genetic predisposition toward overweight and obesity, but it takes considerable, constant effort over a lifetime.

The myth of "spot reducing"

Can you lose weight from one "problem area"?

Contrary to the impression left by many books, videos, and magazine articles, you can't lose weight from one "problem area" exclusively. Spot or area reducing is not possible, because when one loses fat, and hence weight, it is lost proportionally from the entire body. It is impossible to lose weight primarily from the hips, thighs, or abdomen.

Strengthening specific muscle groups, however, is a different question. Poor muscle tone around the abdomen and back usually causes the abdomen to appear fat. The muscles stretch and sag, and then the abdomen sags. Exercises to maintain and increase the strength of the muscles of the back and abdomen will help to prevent and treat most protruding abdomens. The popular "sit-up" is one exercise approach that's effective.

(Note: before undertaking any exercise program, be sure to consult your physician.)

Sit-ups

Lying on your back, with hands crossed behind the neck, knees flexed, rise briskly to a sitting position. This strengthens the back muscles, which are of primary importance in preventing a sagging abdomen. When first starting this simple exercise, some will probably be unable to rise to a sitting position. Initially, then, you might hook your feet under the edge of a bed or heavy chair, and then pull up to a sitting position. After a few months of doing this exercise for 15 to 20 minutes twice a day, muscle strength should be increased sufficiently so that it is not necessary to hook your feet under a heavy object.

While sit-ups represent a good way to develop abdominal muscle tone, other exercises can be helpful in burning off calories as well.

For most people, an exercise program should incorporate some sort of "huffing and puffing" routine. Usually, the objective is to increase your heart rate and get your lungs working harder than usual.

Certainly, there's no shortage of exercise books, articles, and videos you can use to customize your personal fitness program; we offer the following "standbys" as excellent starting points.

Walking or jogging

Jogging is popular these days, but a good brisk walk is also a fine way to bring your calorie expenditure up. Walking is perhaps the simplest and cheapest kind of exercise for most people. (Little-known fact: you'll burn off approximately the same amount of calories—about 100—walking one mile briskly as you will jogging the same distance.) Whether walking or jogging is selected, two sessions of perhaps twenty minutes each per day is a fine target for most of us.

Knee bends

Standing erect, with both arms stretched forward, lower yourself to a squatting position. Then return to a standing position. Repeat the movements slowly; do not force or strain unnecessarily. Beginners may wish to start with a smaller number of knee bends, perhaps fifteen or twenty. Those with more experience may be more ambitious.

Pushups

This is no doubt a familiar exercise for anyone who's served in the armed forces. Lie face down on the floor; place each hand at chest level, about six inches away from the torso. Pushing with your hands and arms only, raise the body in one smooth motion by straightening the arms. Lower the body by bending the arms, touching your nose to the floor. (Optional variation for women: raise only the upper part of the body, leaving the knees in contact with the floor throughout the exercise.) The number of pushups you can do will depend on your current level of upper body strength.

Of course, no one exercise program is right for everyone. Experiment with the above ideas, add some of your own, or consult other sources. Before long, you'll find the balance that's right for you.

A word of caution on the exercises just described—and indeed, on any exercise program. *Do not force yourself to overperform.* Especially if you are beginning an exercise program after a period of comparative inactivity, listen to the messages your body sends you.

If you are in extreme pain after doing 30 pushups, the only thing you will accomplish by attempting 40 will be increasing your chance of injury. Though you shouldn't be afraid to work up a sweat, don't hurt yourself. "No pain, no gain," is a catch-phrase that should never have entered common parlance. A program of modest, steadily more ambitious exercise is preferable to a day or two of exhausting overextension you will not be able to sustain.

Health risks associated with obesity

Is an obese person likely to have a shorter life span than other people?

For most people who are overweight or obese, reaching a reasonable weight is extremely difficult. Yet there are powerful incentives for summoning the reserves of willpower, consistency, and discipline necessary to lose excess body weight through dietary change and a sound exercise program. The fact is simply inescapable: people who are obese carry greater health risks than people who are not. What's more, those risks are interrelated, so that an obese person simultaneously courts a number of serious health hazards, some of which may actually aggravate others.

Heart disease and obesity

How is obesity related to heart disease?

Serum cholesterol levels are slightly higher for obese individuals as a group than for the rest of the population. As we've seen, serum cholesterol levels above 240 mg/dl significantly accelerate the development of plaques in the lining of the blood vessels of the heart. In addition, high blood pressure (itself a serious health problem) is more common in obese individuals, and this definitely accelerates the development of heart disease.

These two factors—plaques and elevated blood pressure—are perhaps the most significant factors associated with obesity that can lead to coronary heart disease (CHD). Add to the latticework of obesity-related CHD risk factors that of diabetes, which, like high blood pressure, is a serious problem in its own right. As these risk factors (and others like smoking, gender, and heredity) mount, the CHD risk becomes greater and greater.

Finally, we must keep in mind that excess body weight is, above and beyond its association with such risk factors, a genuine strain on the heart. After all, the heart has to work harder to push the blood around a body weighing 250 pounds than it does for a body weighing 170 pounds.

Diabetes and obesity

How is obesity related to diabetes?

Obesity, in addition to its other health risks, does contribute to and accelerate the development of diabetes—particularly the diabetes that develops in adults over 35 to 40 years of age.

There are several different types of diabetes, but the two major types are known as juvenile onset and adult onset. Juvenile onset diabetes, as the name implies, develops in childhood and is usually not associated with obesity. Adult onset diabetes usually develops in the late thirties or later and is almost always associated with obesity. In most cases, it disappears when body weight is brought down to a reasonable level.

Diabetes has a strong genetic predisposition. However, if you belong to a family that has experienced problems with the adult-onset variety, keeping your weight at a reasonable level will most likely prevent you from developing this disease.

What do we know about cancer and obesity?

Cancer and obesity

This is one of the many health issues related to obesity where the information is sketchy. Some research suggests that obesity favors the development of cancer of the breast and colon, but the evidence is not, in the opinion of many researchers, conclusive.

In the opinion of the authors, the existing evidence is not strong enough to justify any definitive judgment in this area—other than the general statement that obesity is not conducive to good health. In general, the dietary links with cancer are tenuous ones.

Dangerous diets

Can any diets actually be detrimental to health?

While the widespread interest in calorie consumption, diet, and health topics, is, generally speaking, a positive development, there are several potential hazards to watch out for in the more extreme fad diets.

Some diets, despite the claims of their proponents, can actually injure your health—making their potential for weight reduction, short-term or long-term, something of a secondary issue. Others, such as the currently popular "*8-Week Cholesterol Cure,*" (discussed earlier in this book) not only carry potential health risks (specifically, the overconsumption of niacin, which can result in cirrhosis of the liver) but also substantially misrepresent the existing scientific data. The whole idea of a "cure" for cholesterol is absurd, considering that cholesterol is not a disease in the first place.

Furthermore, no short-term diet has ever been shown to have any lasting effect on serum cholesterol levels. Cholesterol values typically come back to normal within three weeks of returning to normal eating habits. (This is a widely accepted observation within the scientific community; those interested in further information on this much-misrepresented issue are referred to the paper by Schoenfeld, Patsch, Rudel, Nelson, Epstein, and Olson in the May, 1982 issue of *The Journal of Clinical Investigation.*)

"Low calorie" diets

Is losing a great deal of weight in a short period safe?

Any diet of less than 800 to 900 calories, if followed for more than a few weeks, is dangerous to health. This puts many of the "liquid diets" in the hazardous category.

The reason for the increased danger associated with following these diets is simple: with such a limited caloric intake, one will not obtain sufficient nutrients such as protein, vitamins, and minerals.

Dramatic loss of weight will occur with any diet of less than 800 calories, regardless of whether it is liquid or solid in nature. However, the initial pounds lost will be made up mostly of body water, not fat.

Is "water weight" easier to lose than actual body fat?

A pint of water weighs approximately one pound. So water weight, certainly, is a part of excess weight. Many "miracle diets," however, take advantage of the fact that the first few pounds lost on a weight reduction program are mainly made up of water. After that, however, the weight is made up mostly of body fat—and fat is harder to lose.

Whether the excess is water or not, losing weight rapidly (say, three to five pounds a week) is dangerous and may result in faintness, changes in blood pressure, cardiac irregularities, and/or malnutrition. Predictably enough, when one goes off the diet, rapid weight gain almost always takes place.

This weight gain is usually accompanied by an increase in blood cholesterol levels, and an increased development of atherosclerotic deposits in the lining of blood vessels. As a general rule, you should consider these diets a significant risk to your overall health.

(For comparison's sake, consider that a weight loss of one to two pounds a week, for a period of ten to twelve weeks, is typical on a sound diet and exercise program.)[1]

The diet "roller coaster"

Why do people usually gain back the weight they lose?

Why is it so common for a person to lose weight over a short period of time—and then gain it back again?

Part of the answer, of course, has to do with the way we look at food. Eating is one of the pleasures of life, as well as a physiological necessity. If one "starves" on a diet of less than 800 calories for a few weeks, one will lose considerable weight. Shortly thereafter, though, the eagerness for the pleasure of eating is so great that most people return to their former patterns of eating too much and not exercising enough. Not only are the original pounds regained but often extra weight is picked up.

Is there any really dependable way to lose weight—and keep it off?

Unfortunately, where lasting weight loss is concerned, there are usually no quick fixes. The only really dependable way for an overweight or obese person to reach a reasonable weight is to eat less and exercise more—over an extended period.

This way, only one to two pounds are lost per week. Such a pace typically leads to weight loss that can be maintained.

No single food or beverage needs to be eliminated, but it is necessary to decrease the portions of those foods and beverages particularly rich in calories. These foods include meats and whole milk products, particularly ice creams made with whole milk and cream, cheeses, and alcoholic beverages. High-calorie treats such as pies, cakes, pastries, and frozen desserts also fall into this category. Larger portions of foods low in calories, such as salads, fruits, and vegetables, may be eaten in more generous amounts—provided they are not smothered with fatty sauces or dressings.

Can you lose weight and keep it off without exercising?

Remember that an exercise program is a very important part of any weight-loss effort. In fact, it is probably the most important part for most people.

Lifetime changes, not quick fixes

Many dieters think it's possible to lose weight without making long-term, permanent changes in one's diet. In other words, they want to eat "light" for a month as part of a program to lose weight and then return to "normal" eating habits.

Long-range, even lifetime changes in eating and exercise habits are necessary to reach and maintain a reasonable weight—but these changes need not be drastic. After losing five to ten pounds in four or five weeks, you can "coast" for another four to five week period, but don't go back to your previous eating and exercise habits. As soon as you notice a gain of one or two pounds, go back to your new habits for another four or five weeks. Repeat this cycle and before too long your new habits will be your permanent habits!

A suggested meal plan, featuring a modest intake of calories, can be found later in this book. In conjunction with a sound exercise program, it can help many people reach their weight goals.

Chapter Ten: For Women Only

How do nutritional needs of men and women differ?

The dietary needs of both sexes are essentially the same except for the caloric intake, which is usually less for women than for men—because women are usually smaller and less active. In addition, women of childbearing age need more iron because they lose iron during monthly menstrual periods. When menstruation stops after the menopause, a woman's need for iron is similar to that of a man.

Should women consume more dairy foods than men?

One notable difference in recommended dietary guidelines for women as opposed to men, however, is the greater emphasis placed on dairy foods for women—to decrease their chances of problems with osteoporosis. Dairy foods, of course, are excellent sources of calcium, which is necessary for proper bone development and maintenance.

Osteoporosis and dairy products

Osteoporosis is a disease in which the bones become porous due to a loss of calcium. Drinking milk and eating other dairy products is not an absolute prevention for this disease, but it certainly is a great help.

All age groups of females should be generous in consumption of most of the dairy products. Low-fat products, particularly skim milk and cheeses made from it, are good foods for women seeking to lose weight. It is particularly important for women in and beyond the mid-thirties to "institutionalize" the habit of consuming three to four glasses of milk every day.

Pregnancy and breastfeeding

During the first three months of pregnancy, there are no important changes in nutritional requirements for women. During the second trimester, requirements for all nutrients increase a small amount, perhaps five percent. For the last trimester, increases are on the order of ten percent.

Most sources endorse some weight gain (even as much as five pounds) during the first trimester, and substantial gains in the second trimester—perhaps a pound a week. Total weight gain during pregnancy between 20 and 30 pounds is considered to be normal. (Pregnant women, particularly those used to dieting, should note that inadequate weight gain presents risks to the baby and is associated with low birth weight.)

Extra needs of the various nutrients will be obtained if increased food intake is made up of a carefully selected, varied diet from the Basic Four Food Groups.

Intake of milk, skimmed if one is concerned about weight, is usually increased during the second and third trimesters. Many physicians also recommend supplements of iron and folic acid (one of the

B-vitamins) during this period; both nutrients are included in standard prenatal vitamin preparations.

The extra dietary needs of pregnant women should really be decided in each case in consultation with one's physician, not by this or any other book.

What risks are associated with poor diet during pregnancy?

Poor diet during pregnancy: the risks

A low birth weight and various abnormalities of the fetus may arise from poor dietary practices during pregnancy. It is recommended that women eat a good diet during the first month of pregnancy. Unfortunately, it is usually impossible to know if one is pregnant until after the first month menstruation ceases. Though it is certainly true that many women accidentally become pregnant while dieting and experience no problems with fetal development it is fair to say that rigid dieting is not desirable for a month or so before one hopes to become pregnant.

What specific foods should be avoided? Leaving aside for a moment the question of alcohol consumption, there is really nothing in a standard, balanced diet that one must avoid eating or drinking during pregnancy. Occasionally, some pregnant women notice that their ankles and feet begin to swell during pregnancy. In such cases, a woman's doctor may recommend reduction in the intake of salt, which will usually take care of the problem.

Some physicians recommend no intake of alcoholic beverages during pregnancy. This is certainly a safe approach, though perhaps slightly (and understandably) overcautious. At any rate, it probably does not represent advice that every woman can be expected to follow.

What about alcohol consumption during pregnancy?

In 1981, the American Council on Science and Health issued a pamphlet entitled "Alcohol Use During Pregnancy." It contains the following statement: "For those women who choose to drink during pregnancy, ACSH advises that they limit their daily intake to two drinks or less of beer, wine or liquor. The alcoholic content of two 12-ounce glasses of beer, two 4-ounce glasses of table wine, or two mixed drinks each containing 1 1/2 ounces of 80-proof liquor is approximately the same: each contains about one ounce of 100 percent alcohol."

No absolutely safe level of alcohol consumption during pregnancy has ever been defined except total abstinence. There are substantial differences among all women (and, for that matter, among all people) in their ability to tolerate alcohol. The safest course, then, and the one many women select, is to avoid alcohol entirely during pregnancy—particularly during the first one or two months.

Formula vs. breastfeeding

Which is preferable for a baby: breast milk or formula?

Breastfeeding is definitely preferable to formula feeding for both nutritional and psychological reasons.

Breast milk from a healthy, well-nourished mother provides an optimal source of nutrition for most infants. It is inexpensive, contains disease-resistance factors, and does not stress the infant's immature organ system. Commercially prepared formulas can and do play an important role in infant nutrition in technologically advanced countries but are an imperfect permanent substitute for mother's milk.

Breastfeeding is generally pleasant for both the mother and infant and encourages close, affectionate contact that may enhance bonding. Most pediatricians endorse breastfeeding through the first six months of a baby's life, and some mothers nurse even longer.

When breastfeeding is insufficient, inappropriate, or discontinued early, commercially-prepared formulas serve as a valuable nutritional supplement or as an effective alternative to breast milk.

Breastfeeding women, like other adults, should eat a varied, balanced diet selected from the Basic Four Food Groups, but with an increase of caloric intake of perhaps 30 percent. (Breastfeeding requires energy—hence the need for the extra calories.) In addition, they should increase by approximately 20 percent their intake of protein, vitamins, and minerals. This means, in essence, perhaps one more serving of high-protein foods such as meats or legumes, and an extra serving of vegetables, compared to a standard diet for an adult female. An additional glass or two of milk—to bring daily intake to four glasses a day—is also recommended.

If the mother cannot consume this quantity of milk, a calcium supplement supplying approximately one gram of calcium daily is an idea that should be discussed with one's physician.

What are anorexia nervosa and bulimia?

Eating disorders associated primarily with women

Two related eating disorders have been topics of much discussion in recent years: anorexia nervosa and bulimia. Sufferers of each disorder are usually adolescent girls and young women. The medical risks associated with anorexia nervosa and bulimia can be quite serious.

Anorexia nervosa (literally, "nervous loss of appetite") has been described as "self-starvation from a morbid fear of obesity." It usually begins when a girl of normal weight or slightly above normal weight begins a diet, reaches the target weight, but does not return to normal eating habits. Even emaciated anorexia nervosa victims still consider themselves obese. It's estimated that as many as 10 percent of all adolescent girls develop anorexia nervosa; of that number, 9 percent starve themselves to death, and 2 to 5 percent commit suicide.

Physical changes associated with this disease include the cessation of the menstrual cycle, cardiac irregularities, and difficulties in adapting to temperature change.

Bulimia, or "binging," is a disorder in which sufferers (usually, women between the ages of 17 and 25) consume very large amounts of food and deliberately bring about vomiting to avoid weight gain. Bulimics, like anorexics, are obsessively concerned with diet and body weight issues; however, bulimics virtually always recognize this compulsive behavior for what it is and are concerned about it.

Repeated vomiting can have detrimental effects on the function of the digestive tract and may lower levels of essential nutrients in the body, notably potassium. Abuse of diuretics, laxatives, and vomit-inducing preparations is common among bulimics; such abuse presents a number of serious health hazards.

The exact causes of these disorders are not known, but current thinking is that both are primarily psychiatric problems. Cultural and sociological pressures may play a role, as well; sufferers are typically from middle-class or upper-middle-class households.

Anorexia nervosa and bulimia represent serious health risks; qualified medical and psychiatric help is strongly advised if any of the above signs present themselves.

Chapter Eleven: Eating Right in a Complicated World

The Basic Four

What are the Basic Four Food Groups?

The Basic Four Food Groups were developed by Harvard's Department of Nutrition in the early 1950s, presented at the Annual Meeting of the American Dietetic Association in May of 1955, and published in the November 1955 issue of the *Journal of the American Dietetic Association*. They were developed (under Dr. Stare's chairmanship at Harvard's Department of Nutrition) in an attempt to simplify the teaching of practical nutrition by dividing most of our common foods into four groups.

The guidelines still represent perhaps the most important nutritional advice for most Americans. If you eat a reasonable quantity of some foods each day from each of the Basic Four Food Groups, you will probably receive adequate amounts of all the known nutrients.

The Basic Four Food Groups are: fruits and vegetables; enriched or whole grain cereals, products made from them, and potatoes; milk and products made from milk, such as cheeses and ice creams; and meat, poultry, fish, eggs, and legumes.

In 1957, the Department of Agriculture also published what they called the Basic Four Food Groups; they were the same as those developed at Harvard. The Basic Four, as they are commonly called, are by far the most widely used teaching tool for nutrition.

THE BASIC FOUR FOOD GROUPS

Fruits and vegetables

To obtain vitamins, minerals, and fiber (also known as "roughage"), most people are advised to eat four servings from this group daily. Citrus fruits or tomatoes should be included at least once a day; dark green or yellow vegetables should be included at least four times over the course of a week.

Bread and cereal products

Whole-grain or enriched bread and cereals, grain-based products such as pasta, and potatoes are included in this group. Such foods supply carbohydrates, vitamins, minerals, and some protein. Four or more servings from this group per day are recommended for most people.

Dairy products

Milk, one of the most important of all foods in our diet, heads the list here. Virtually all adults and children should consume some milk or milk product every day. Milk and foods made from milk provide calcium, protein, vitamins, and carbohydrates. As a general rule, cheese, ice cream, yogurt, and other foods made from milk are good occasional substitutes for liquid milk. Two to four glasses of milk per day are usually recommended for most people; pregnant and nursing mothers need somewhat more.

Meat or meat substitutes

Fish, eggs, poultry, beans and peas (legumes), and nuts, in addition to meat, make up this group. Two servings every day from the meat or meat substitute group will supply protein, iron, and some important vitamins.

No such thing as perfect food

Why is it important to eat foods from these groups?

Why is it important to eat according to these guidelines? Because no single food contains all of the 50 or more nutrients so far identified.

For example, fruits are good sources of most of the water-soluble vitamins (particularly vitamin C), minerals, and fiber, but have essentially no protein.

Vegetables are good sources of minerals, fiber, and some vitamins, but the protein is low in both quantity and quality. The green and yellow vegetables are good sources of carotenes, some of which are converted into vitamin A in the liver and other body tissues.

Milk and its related products are by far the best sources of calcium; they also provide good quality protein and many of the vitamins, but are low in iron and in vitamin C.

The meat group provides iron that is readily absorbed, other minerals, many vitamins, and protein of high nutritional quality, but does not offer, for instance, much calcium. Legumes, such as peas and beans, are included in the meat group because of their protein. They are also good sources of fiber.

Grains, breads, and cereals are important sources of protein, carbohydrate, and the B-vitamins, particularly thiamin and niacin. However, they do not provide significant amounts of calcium, vitamin C, or a number of other important nutrients.

In order to obtain all of the nutrients in adequate amounts, one must eat a variety of foods from among and within each of the Basic Four.

The term "among and within" probably deserves some elaboration. For the sake of variety and to insure an exposure to a broad range of nutrients, nutritionists recommend that people use the Basic Four judiciously—and avoid, for instance, eating only potatoes from the cereal and grain group for weeks on end. Fortunately, people usually don't need much persuading on this score. As long as you eat a varied diet, the Basic Four represents an excellent way to choose balanced food combinations for any given day.

Of course, selecting the foods isn't the only choice to make. The size of servings, particularly of those foods containing generous amounts of fats, must be adjusted to a person's energy expenditure, so that the body grows properly and reaches and maintains a reasonable weight.

Over the long term—months or years—all nutrients are essential for health. However, it is not necessary to obtain all nutrients every day, because we have the capacity to store many nutrients in various tissues of the body.

Must I consume all the nutrients every day?

For example, calcium is stored in bones, vitamin A and D in the liver, and amino acids can be stored in many body tissues, particularly muscle tissue. In general, we are able to store fat-soluble nutrients in body fat but we are only able to store water-soluble nutrients for a short length of time, only a few weeks at the most.

As we're all aware, people are also able to store fat—but often too much of it, and in parts of the body that are quite evident!

Recommended Dietary Allowances

What is the "R.D.A."? The "U.S.R.D.A."?

The Recommended Dietary Allowances, or R.D.A.s, were devised by the Food and Nutrition Board of the National Research Council and are recommended levels of various nutrients for daily consumption. They were first established in 1943 and, on the basis of continuing research, have been slightly revised about every five years. The last published revision was in 1980 and was the ninth revision.

The R.D.A.s are not requirements for individuals but rather recommendations for the average daily amounts of certain nutrients that healthy population groups should consume over a period of time. They are set at levels estimated to exceed the actual requirements (except for calories) of most individuals. They thereby ensure that the nutritional needs of nearly all members of all populations will be met if the guidelines are followed.

The U.S.R.D.A. (U.S. Recommended Daily Allowance) is a standard similar to the R.D.A.s. These levels were established by the Food and Drug Administration in 1974, are patterned after the R.D.A.s, and serve as the basis for the nutrition labeling of foods. They have not been revised since they were formulated.

If someone regularly eats less than the R.D.A., does that mean the person is malnourished?

Intakes below the R.D.A. for a nutrient are not necessarily inadequate. Remember, these government and scientific guidelines are not requirements, but recommended nutrient intakes for healthy populations. They are also set at levels appreciably higher than most people's requirements and can be readily obtained from diets comprised of food selections from each of the Basic Four.

Of vitamins and vitamin supplements

A major breach in meaning has occurred, over the years, in most discussions about food and nutrition. It is this: when we say "vitamin," we are often referring to a pill that comes in a little bottle from a supermarket, drug store, or health food store. Actually these pills (and their related products) are *vitamin supplements*—and should be referred to as such, because *vitamins* are the organic substances found in food (though sometimes also produced synthetically) that are essential to normal, healthy life. Referring to the supplements as "vitamins," while technically accurate, gives the impression that the average person could forego the vitamins in the food in favor of the pills—and this is not so.

Vitamin supplements are certainly *not* essential to good health—but vitamins are.

Are vitamin supplements essential to good health?

Vitamins are substances that have a very specific definition. Nutritionists and scientists consider a vitamin to be an organic compound that is needed in very small quantities in the diet to promote growth and maintain life. The "very small quantities" provision keeps carbohydrates, fats, or protein from being classified as vitamins.

A substance that is a vitamin for humans may not be a vitamin for some other animals. For example, ascorbic acid (known to most of us as vitamin C) is a vitamin for humans, monkeys, and guinea pigs—but not for rats, who can synthesize it themselves and don't need it in the diet.

There are thirteen known vitamins for humans. They are divided into two categories: water-soluble and fat-soluble. The water-soluble vitamins are usually not stored by the body for any longer than a few weeks. The fat-soluble vitamins, on the other hand, can be retained for months.

WATER-SOLUBLE VITAMINS

B-vitamins:
thiamin, riboflavin, niacin, pantothenic acid, folacin, pyridoxine (vitamin B_6), biotin, and cobalamine (vitamin B_{12})

vitamin C

FAT-SOLUBLE VITAMINS

vitamin A
vitamin D
vitamin E
vitamin K

Many vitamins function as catalysts—substances that initiate or speed up chemical reactions but remain unchanged while performing their tasks repeatedly. This explains why only tiny amounts are needed in the diet.

Vitamins themselves do not provide energy. Many are part of enzyme systems required for the release of energy from carbohydrates, fats, protein, or alcohol, the only sources of energy we have. Normal growth and maintenance of body tissues depends on an adequate supply of all the vitamins.

Vitamins were first isolated from various foods during the early part of this century, but by now they have all been produced in the laboratory. There is no difference in structure or function between naturally occurring vitamins in food and those that are manmade and generally contained in vitamin supplements. As Gertrude Stein might put it, a vitamin is a vitamin is a vitamin. The crucial question is not whether the supplements function properly but whether or not you need them in the first place!

As noted earlier, the main source for vitamins should be the food we eat. In a balanced diet, it is unnecessary to rely on the synthesized or heavily processed products that are thought, somewhat ironically, to be part of the stable of "health food" products. For those who profess to abstain from "processed foods," the decision to take large amounts of vitamin supplements is a strange one. Vitamin supplements probably represent the most heavily processed food-related products available to consumers.

Vitamin supplements do, however, provide vitamins more or less as advertised. One vitamin product generally supplies more than one type, but usually not all of the available vitamins.

Will taking vitamin supplements compensate for a poor diet?

Taking vitamin supplements as part of an unsatisfactory diet will not result in good nutrition—unless the diet is poor in that particular vitamin or vitamins. This is seldom the case if one consumes a daily diet selected from among and within each of the Basic Four Food Groups.

Actually, there are very few circumstances where anyone's health can be improved by taking vitamin supplements. If one is convalescing from an illness in which considerable body weight has been lost, or an illness in which food was poorly absorbed, taking a multivitamin supplement for a few weeks may be helpful. In addition, pregnant or nursing mothers may be advised to increase their intake of certain vitamins and/or minerals. It's important to point out, however, that such situations involve issues that must be resolved through discussions with a physician, not independently in a supermarket checkout line.

Vitamin supplements, like many other preparations, may provide a strong (and favorable) psychological effect. Beyond that, many nutritionists agree, their value is negligible for most people.

Except when used as part of the treatment of a disease, vitamin supplements should be used to provide no more than the levels suggested by the R.D.A.s for a given nutrient. Remember, most of us receive adequate amounts of vitamins from a varied diet.

Will taking vitamin supplements make one feel more energetic?

Contrary to popular belief, taking vitamin supplements will have no measurable effect on your overall energy level—unless your diet has been woefully inadequate for some time and you are, as a result, suffering from severe malnourishment. Again, in this case, the advice of a physician is essential.

If all the above seems new to you, that's probably because most Americans have come to believe that ingesting vitamin supplements in any dosage is good for you—and that ingesting large doses must therefore be *extremely* good for you. In most cases, this is untrue.

Can you take too many vitamins?

You *can* take too many vitamins—and many people do. Large-scale consumption of some vitamins, notably the water-soluble vitamin C, is harmless. With vitamin C, excesses are readily excreted with the urine; the same is true of many of the B-vitamins. The fat soluble vitamins, though, particularly A and D, can cause health problems when taken in amounts five to ten times the Recommended Dietary Allowance levels for a period of a month or more.

Minerals

Minerals, unlike vitamins, are inorganic—they contain no carbon. Like vitamins, however, they often act as catalysts for the release of energy from carbohydrates, fats, and proteins. Minerals are also available commercially as supplements.

Some 21 minerals are now considered essential for humans, including iron, calcium, potassium, and others. Sodium, too, is a mineral—one Americans tend to consume too heavily.

Should I reduce my sodium intake?

Reducing sodium intake (usually through decreasing use of salt) is generally recognized as a good dietary goal for most Americans. That having been said, the same general principles apply here as with vitamin supplements. What you need, you should be able to obtain from your diet. Though minerals, too, can be used in the treatment of some physical disorders, they should only be used in this way under the advice of a physician. Like vitamins, some minerals can be harmful if taken in excessive amounts.

One final note on vitamin and mineral supplements. All three authors of this book manage to get by without them, as do all their children and (in the cases of Drs. Stare and Olson) grandchildren!

How much liquid should we drink?

A great deal of emphasis is placed on what we eat, but less attention is paid to what we *drink*. Of course, the health risks associated with alcohol are well known. But what about normal, daily consumption of fluids?

Thirst is usually a good indicator of how much liquid to drink, but the liquid need not be water. We really mean fluid, which can be fruit juice, soft drinks, coffee, tea, milk, etc. A more scientific way to recommend fluid intake is to consume enough fluid to excrete one and a half to two quarts of urine in each 24 hours.

For practical purposes, this requires drinking about six to eight eight-ounce servings of fluid in each 24 hour period. In addition to losing water via urine, water is lost with fecal wastes, in the breath, and in perspiration.

Are soft drinks an acceptable substitute for water?

Drinking colas and other soft drinks is an acceptable substitute for drinking equal quantities of water if the extra calories are not a problem for you.

Consumption of soft drinks has increased in recent years but has replaced drinking water more than it has replaced the consumption of other nutritionally important liquids like milk.

If consumption of soft drinks appreciably decreases the intake of milk, nutritional health will be adversely affected. All of us should have at least two to three glasses of milk each day; fluid intake beyond that can be of your choice and can include soft drinks.

What health problems are associated with caffeine?

Many people express concern at the health implications of beverages that contain caffeine, notably soft drinks, coffee, and tea. It seems appropriate here to quote from *The Health Effects of Caffeine*, a publication of the American Council on Science and Health:

"Caffeine as generally consumed in foods, beverages, and over the counter drugs is not a threat to the health of most Americans. However, some people who consume large amounts of products that contain caffeine may experience health problems, including chronic headaches, sleep disturbances, rapid heart beat, anxiety, stomach upset, and depression. . . . Consumers should recognize that caffeine is a drug with potent stimulant properties. These stimulant effects vary from person to person and sensitive individuals should be particularly cautious about its use."

In addition, consumers should note recent research on the subject of caffeine as it relates to smoking. An article in the April 22, 1989 issue of the *British Medical Journal* suggests that smokers metabolize caffeine abnormally rapidly but that this effect disappears quickly after one stops smoking. Therefore, the article suggests, if a person quits smoking and maintains his previous caffeine consumption level, the caffeine concentration in the blood more than doubles. The resulting symptoms may contribute to the jumpiness that is part of tobacco withdrawal.

Chapter Twelve: Food on the Run

Short on time?

In the abstract, it sounds easy enough to eat a sensible diet. All one has to do is plan meals that include a variety of foods from among and within the Basic Four Food Groups. But for many of us, there is little time to shop and prepare meals.

Considering the rise of the two-career family, and our increased reliance on convenience foods such as frozen and microwaveable meals, fast food, and heavily processed "instant" preparations, a discussion of the nutritional aspects of these foods seems appropriate.

Are processed foods lower in nutrients than other foods?

In the first place, consumers should know that such processed foods do not represent substantial losses in nutritional quality.

Unless, in processing, fats or carbohydrates are added, prepared foods are roughly equal to fresh food products in terms of calories. Such additions are, however, quite common, and consumers should check ingredient lists carefully.

For example, in canned vegetables and fruits, a small amount of sugar is usually added to improve flavor. This addition increases the caloric content of the food. However, if the same sweetener, in the same amount, is added to fresh vegetables or fruits when prepared, the same effect on caloric content of the food occurs.

Microwave ovens

Contrary to what many suspect, a microwave oven does nothing whatsoever to impair the nutritional quality of the foods prepared in it. Nor do these ovens, when properly used, present any health risks to the general population.

Microwave ovens are a great convenience for those who have little time to spend in the kitchen. Products designed for preparation in these devices represent substantial advances in food technology. There is no harmful residual irradiation associated with these products—using and eating food properly cooked in microwave ovens is not dangerous to consumers in any way.

Are any dangers associated with microwave ovens?

Can use of microwave ovens be dangerous? Certainly—just as a conventional oven, a blender, or a set of kitchen knives can. Foods that are cooked in some sealed containers in a microwave oven can explode; foods that are not sufficiently cooked can contain harmful bacteria; overheated foods can burn your mouth. People with infants should resist the temptation to heat up bottles of baby formula in the microwave oven, as this is extremely dangerous. Formula heated in this way may be tepid in one part of the bottle but scalding elsewhere. The only way a parent would know about any potential injury would be the baby's scream—and by then, of course, it would be too late.

With simple precautions and a little common sense, however, a microwave oven is a safe and useful household tool.

"Microwave meals"

So much for the equipment. Now, how solid nutritionally is a diet that includes generous helpings of "microwave meals"?

Such a diet needn't be a problem. Think for a moment about what frozen meals usually contain. Typically, there's a serving of meat, chicken, or fish; a modest portion of a green or yellow vegetable; and rice or potatoes.

What's missing? Milk. In addition, you might want to increase the intake from the fruit and vegetable group—perhaps by supplementing the meal with a pear or banana for dessert.

A meal planned around microwave pizza topped with pepperoni, using the same approach, would simply need more vegetables—a spinach salad, for instance. (The pepperoni reflects the meat group, while the dairy and cereal groups are represented by the cheese and crust of the pizza, respectively.)

Note that a cheeseburger on an enriched bun with lettuce and tomato, whether prepared with a microwave or purchased at a fast food restaurant, does deliver something from each of the Basic

Four Food Groups. As a general rule, occasional consumption of this popular food, perhaps bolstered by a serving of milk, certainly poses no nutritional risk—though it is somewhat higher in fat than other foods you could select.

Intelligent choices

Fast food, frozen meals, and other convenience foods are often generous in salt and fats, which is one reason they should be selected carefully if they represent more than an occasional part of your diet. The salt problem, logically enough, can be addressed by simply avoiding table salt altogether when eating these foods. As for the fat, you can usually gauge this with foods bought in the supermarket by checking the total calories per serving and comparing it to other products. (See the section on food labeling later in this chapter.)

Many fast food restaurants and supermarkets now feature salad bars, adding a new twist to the whole idea of convenience foods. This development has made it easy for consumers in a hurry to obtain good-quality servings of fresh fruits and vegetables.

How do "light" versions of popular foods compare to other foods?

While we're on the subject of processed foods, we should touch on the much-ballyhooed marketing phenomenon of "light" foods.

There is still no F.D.A. regulation with regard to what calorie reduction is required in order to call a product "light"—whether it is beer, salad dressing, or anything else. The phrase as used certainly implies fewer calories, but how many fewer calories, and compared to what, is very much open to question. As of this writing, you could, theoretically, market your own brand of "Special Light Lard" without making any adjustments in the product's calorie content.

Our guess is that it makes very little difference in regard to one's total caloric intake whether one consumes "light" food products rather than "heavy" equivalents.

Labeling

What labeling guidelines must food producers follow?

Basically there are two kinds of labeling of prepared foods—ingredient listings and nutritional information.

Ingredient listing is, as the name implies, a list of the major ingredients of the food. These are listed in descending order of the amount of the item in the product. For example, a salad dressing label might list ingredients as follows: water, vinegar, soybean oil, corn syrup, salt, onion, garlic, monosodium glutamate, and artificial colorings. This product would contain more water than anything else.

In addition to ingredient listing, a product must carry certain nutritional information if any nutritional claims are made, and this information must appear in a prescribed format. Each nutritional label must have the following information:

NUTRITIONAL LABELING REQUIREMENTS

Serving size for which the nutrition information is given.

Number of servings in the container.

Number of calories per serving.

Grams of protein per serving.

Grams of carbohydrate per serving.

Grams of fat per serving.

Milligrams of sodium per serving.

Percentages of the U.S. Recommended Daily Allowance for protein, vitamin A, vitamin C, thiamin, riboflavin, niacin, calcium, and iron provided by the size serving. (The label must state whether any of these are less than two percent of U.S.R.D.A. levels for a given nutrient.)

Nutrition information does not have to be restricted to the listing of the above nutrients. Twelve additional vitamins and minerals have U.S.R.D.A. values, and the nutritional contribution of a food toward these values also may be provided if a manufacturer wishes to do so.

As an aid to individuals on special diets, a few products are labeled with the level of cholesterol contained in a serving. (For instance, the salad dressing we took as an example might feature a line in the nutritional summary describing a cholesterol content of zero—and could claim on its front label to be "cholesterol free." Similarly, persons on a sodium (salt) restricted diet may be interested in the sodium content of a given product.

Traditionally, some foods are eaten with another food added rather than being eaten alone. Therefore, a second column of nutrition information may be presented to show the contribution of the food combination as it is eaten. Such a listing, for example, is usually provided for breakfast cereals plus milk.

Remember, it is necessary to consider the calories and nutrients in the total food and beverage intake and not merely rely on labeled foods for information. Fresh fruits, vegetables, and meats are excellent sources of many nutrients, but their contributions are not identified in the clear-cut manner required for many processed foods.

This inconsistency could be addressed with a minimal change in the current guidelines for processed foods. Any label concerning nutrition might also carry a phrase like "To be well nourished, eat a variety of foods from the Basic Four Food Groups."

Variety and moderation

It is easy to eat a balanced diet, even if you eat convenience foods or fast foods with some frequency—assuming you use a little common sense. No matter where you are or what you eat, remember that variety and moderation (in a word, "balance") are the watchwords for sound nutrition.

"Skipping breakfast"

Is skipping breakfast dangerous?

Do you rush out the door for work in the morning without eating—and eat something to "tide you over" (such as a sweet roll, a cup of coffee, or a doughnut) from a lunch truck or take-out window later on?

These habits are not dangerous if they don't represent a daily practice, but they are usually not helpful in promoting intelligent daily food selection and good long-term nutrition. Most people wake up hungry in the morning. They should take the body's hint and have some breakfast.

When you consider that most of us consume our dinner around seven p.m., making the body wait till noon of the following day for something substantial is a little extreme. A doughnut or sweet roll with a cup of coffee is certainly not substantial from a nutritional standpoint, and shouldn't be incorporated into your daily routine as a standard breakfast.

Why not substitute some cereal with milk and a piece of fruit? (It won't take *that* long.) Occasionally, when you have a few extra minutes, you might even opt for some juice, toast or a muffin with some butter or cheese, and an egg and a couple of strips of bacon or sausage. (While we cannot appeal to any scientific studies that may exist on the question, the authors have a strong suspicion that getting up early enough to prepare a good breakfast has more to do with willpower than a person's physical need for sleep.)

Breakfast is an important meal that should, for most of us, be on the generous side. If any meal is to be diminished in order to keep body weight at a reasonable level, we suggest it be lunch or dinner.

Better still, engage in more physical activity to burn up those calories that are so pleasant to consume!

Meal elimination to lose weight

Is it advisable to skip a meal routinely to try to lose weight?

By the way, the common habit of skipping a meal (usually breakfast) for weight-loss purposes is almost always futile. One becomes so hungry later in the day that there is tremendous temptation to overeat at the next meal—and to snack continuously (or "graze," to use a currently popular term) throughout the day.

Replenishing your food intake three times a day, but with modest amounts at either midday or evening, is the best reduction plan to follow. In addition, of course, sufficient exercise is a crucial component of a weight-loss program, especially when combined with a reduction of foods rich in fat and with moderate (if any) consumption of alcoholic beverages. (Beer, wine, and spirits are high in calories and provide virtually no nutrients.) As we have learned in this chapter, a balanced diet can incorporate processed or "instant" food products. With judicious selection and common sense when it comes to serving sizes and calorie intakes, such foods can be part of a sensible weight-loss plan as well.

Chapter Thirteen: Day by Day

The Basic Four

This chapter outlines suggested menus for seven consecutive days for adults who wish to maintain their current weight, as well as for those interested in losing weight. The diets are based on a balanced diet selected from among and within the Basic Four Food Groups.

The Basic Four Food Groups

Fruits and vegetables

Cereals and foods made from them, and potatoes

Milk and related products

Meat and meat alternatives

While the menus are designed for use by adults, the guidelines that follow can be readily adapted to children, adolescents, and senior citizens, mainly by adjusting portion sizes—particularly of foods in the meat and milk group.

Intake of milk should be increased by, say, 25%-50% for growing children, women who are pregnant or lactating, women over approximately 35 years of age, and senior citizens.

Most people today are concerned about reducing intakes of fats, oils, and sugar. The following diet is modest in these areas—but hardly draconian.

As for alcoholic beverages, they have not been included, but can, in moderation, certainly be part of a healthy diet for adults and senior citizens. One to two servings of alcoholic beverage daily is a good maximum level for most of us. Pregnant women, wary of the potential for fetal damage as a result of excess alcohol consumption, often decide to abstain from alcohol entirely during pregnancy.

There are four diets in this chapter: male maintenance, male reduction, female maintenance, and female reduction. Combined with a sensible exercise program, the diets set out here can help you reach or stay at a reasonable weight. You may wish to consult a physician before deciding to limit your calorie intake further. Remember, diets that are too low in calories—below 800 calories per day for most adults—can be hazardous to your health.

SEVEN-DAY MEAL PLAN FOR . . .

. . . MOST ADULT MALES

who wish to MAINTAIN their current weight (approximately 2200 calories daily)

DAY ONE

Breakfast

1/2 cup orange juice
3/4 cup ready-to-eat cereal
1 cup 1% low-fat milk
1/2 cup fruit
1 slice whole wheat toast
1 teaspoon margarine
coffee or tea

Lunch

Peanut butter and jelly sandwich with 3 tablespoons peanut butter and 2 tablespoons jelly
Apple
8 oz. 1% low-fat milk

Snack

1 cup low-fat yogurt

Dinner

4 oz. filet of haddock, pan-browned with 2 teaspoons margarine
Tossed salad with 2 tablespoons low-cal dressing
1/2 cup steamed fresh broccoli with lemon and 1 teaspoon margarine
1/2 cup macaroni and cheese, prepared with skim milk and margarine
1 cup fruit salad
Coffee or tea

DAY TWO

Breakfast

1/2 cup grapefruit juice
1 poached egg
2 slices whole wheat toast
2 teaspoons butter or margarine
8 oz. 1% low-fat milk
Coffee or tea

Lunch

2 oz. grilled cheese sandwich on whole wheat bread, grilled with 1 teaspoon margarine
1 oz. potato chips (approx. 15 chips)
Orange
8 oz. 1% low-fat milk

Snack

2 cups popcorn (air-popped or microwaved)
8 oz. 1% low-fat milk

Dinner

Tossed lettuce and tomato salad with 2 tablespoons low-cal French dressing
2 slices roast beef (approx. 4 oz.)
3/4 cup mashed potatoes
2 teaspoons margarine
1 cup fresh zucchini sauteed with onion
Dinner roll
Coffee or tea

DAY THREE

Breakfast

1/4 cantaloupe melon (or: 4 oz. orange juice)
3/4 cup oatmeal (instant or quick)
8 oz. 1% low-fat milk
1 slice whole wheat toast
2 teaspoons margarine
1 tablespoon jelly
Coffee or tea

Lunch

Tuna salad sandwich on roll (approx. 3/4 cup tuna, 3 teaspoons mayonnaise)
3 tomato wedges
Apple
8 oz. 1% low-fat milk

Snack

1 oz. cheese
3 saltine crackers
8 oz. iced tea (or: a soft drink)

Dinner

4 oz. broiled breast of chicken
Tossed salad with 1 tablespoon oil and vinegar dressing
Baked potato (approx. 2 1/2 × 4 3/4″)
2 teaspoons margarine
3/4 cup steamed broccoli with lemon
8 oz. 1% low-fat milk
1/2 cup vanilla ice cream
Coffee or tea

DAY FOUR

Breakfast

4 oz. orange juice
3/4 cup ready-to-eat cereal
1/2 cup fruit
1 cup 1% low-fat milk
1 slice whole wheat toast
2 teaspoons margarine
1 tablespoon jam
Coffee or tea

Lunch

3 oz. sliced chicken sandwich on whole wheat bread with lettuce, tomato, and 2 teaspoons mayonnaise
1/2 cup fruit
Coffee, tea, or low-fat milk

Snack

1/4 cup shelled almonds (approximately 40)
Soft drink

Dinner

Tossed salad with 1 tablespoon oil and vinegar dressing
3 oz. broiled pork chop
1 cup cooked rice
1 teaspoon margarine
1/2 cup applesauce
1/2 cup cooked fresh green beans
8 oz. 1% low-fat milk (or: coffee or tea)

DAY FIVE

Breakfast

4 oz. orange juice
2 slices French toast with 1/4 cup maple syrup (4 tablespoons)
8 oz. 1% low-fat milk
Coffee or tea

Lunch

3/4 cup cottage cheese with 2 pineapple rings on lettuce
2 bread sticks (4″ long)
1 cup vegetable soup
8 oz. 1% low-fat milk

Snack

2 cups popcorn (air-popped or microwaved)
8 oz. juice (or: a soft drink)

Dinner

Tossed salad with 1 tablespoon oil and vinegar dressing
4 oz. flounder sauteed with 2 teaspoons margarine
1/2 cup cook beets
1/2 cup steamed cauliflower with 1 teaspoon margarine
1/2 cup spinach noodles with 2 teaspoons margarine
Coffee or tea

DAY SIX

Breakfast

4 oz. orange juice
3/4 cup cooked cereal
1 cup low-fat milk
1 slice whole wheat toast
2 teaspoons margarine
1 tablespoon jam
Coffee or tea

Lunch

3 oz. Virginia ham sandwich on rye bread, with lettuce, tomato, and 1 teaspoon mayonnaise
Apple
8 oz. 1% low-fat milk

Snack

8 oz. low-fat yogurt
1/2 banana

Dinner

Tossed salad with 1 tablespoon low-fat French dressing
4 oz. broiled steak
1/2 cup sauteed mushrooms
Baked potato (approx. 2 1/2″ *x* 4 3/4″)
2 teaspoons margarine
4 steamed asparagus spears
1 cup fresh fruit salad
8 oz. 1% low-fat milk (or: coffee or tea)

DAY SEVEN

Breakfast

4 oz. stewed apricots
1 scrambled egg
1 toasted bagel
2 teaspoons butter or margarine
1 tablespoon jelly
8 oz. 1% low-fat milk
Coffee or tea

Lunch

3 oz. turkey sandwich on whole wheat bread, with lettuce, tomato, and 1 teaspoon mayonnaise
Piece of fruit (or: 1/2 cup fruit)
8 oz. 1% low-fat milk

Snack

2 cookies
8 oz. 1% low-fat milk

Dinner

Tossed salad with 1 tablespoon oil and vinegar dressing
2 slices lean roast pork loin (approx. 4 oz)
3/4 cup oven-browned potatoes
1/2 cup peas with 1 teaspoon margarine
1/2 cup sweetened applesauce
8 oz. 1% low-fat milk (or: coffee or tea)
1/2 cup strawberries, topped with 1/4 cup low-fat yogurt or ice cream

SEVEN-DAY MEAL PLAN FOR . . .

. . . MOST ADULT MALES

who wish to REDUCE their current weight (approximately 1800 calories daily)

DAY ONE

Breakfast

1/2 cup orange juice
3/4 cup ready-to-eat cereal
8 oz. skim milk
3-4 stewed prunes
1 slice whole wheat toast
1 teaspoon margarine
Coffee or tea (sugar-free)

Lunch

Peanut butter and jelly sandwich with 2 tablespoons peanut butter and 1 tablespoon jelly
Apple
8 oz. skim milk

Snack

1 cup low-fat yogurt

Dinner

4 oz. filet of haddock, pan-browned with 2 teaspoons margarine
Tossed salad, with 2 tablespoons low-cal dressing
1/2 cup steamed fresh broccoli with lemon
1/2 small baked potato, with 1 teaspoon margarine
1 cup fruit salad
Coffee or tea (sugar-free)

DAY TWO

Breakfast

1/2 cup grapefruit juice
1/2 banana
3/4 cup ready-to-eat cereal
1 piece dry whole wheat toast
1 cup 1% low-fat milk
Coffee or tea (sugar-free)

Lunch

2 oz. grilled cheese sandwich on whole wheat bread, grilled with 1 teaspoon margarine
Orange
8 oz. skim milk

Snack

2 cups popcorn (air-popped or microwaved)
Diet soft drink

Dinner

Tossed lettuce and tomato salad with 2 tablespoons low-cal French dressing
2 slices roast beef (approx. 4 oz.)
3/4 cup mashed potatoes
2 teaspoons margarine
1 cup fresh zucchini, sauteed with onion
Dinner roll
8 oz. skim milk (or: coffee or tea , sugar-free)

DAY THREE

Breakfast

1/4 cantaloupe melon (or: other fruit)
3/4 cup cooked cereal (instant or quick)
1 cup 1% low-fat milk
1 slice whole wheat toast
1 teaspoon butter or margarine
Coffee or tea (sugar-free)

Lunch

Tuna salad sandwich on roll (approx. 3/4 cup tuna, 2 teaspoons mayonnaise)
3 tomato wedges
Apple
8 oz. skim milk

Snack

1 oz. cheese

3 saltine crackers

8 oz. iced tea (sugar-free) (or: diet soft drink)

Dinner

3 oz. broiled breast of chicken

Tossed salad with 1 tablespoon oil and vinegar dressing

Baked potato (approx. 2 1/2 × 4 3/4″)

1 teaspoon margarine

3/4 cup steamed broccoli with lemon and parsley

8 oz. skim milk

DAY FOUR

Breakfast

4 oz. orange or other juice
3/4 cup ready-to-eat cereal
1/2 cup fresh fruit
1 cup skim milk
1 slice whole wheat toast
1 teaspoon margarine
Coffee or tea (sugar-free)

Lunch

3 oz. sliced chicken sandwich on whole wheat bread with lettuce, tomato, and 2 teaspoons mayonnaise
Fruit
8 oz. skim milk

Snack

1/8 cup shelled almonds (approx. 20)
Diet soft drink

Dinner

Tossed salad, with 1 tablespoon oil and vinegar dressing
3 oz. broiled pork chop
1/2 cup cooked rice
1 teaspoon margarine
1/2 cup applesauce
8 oz. skim milk

DAY FIVE

Breakfast

4 oz. orange juice
2 slices French toast, with diet syrup
8 oz. skim milk
Coffee or tea (sugar-free)

Lunch

1/2 cup cottage cheese, with fruit on lettuce
2 bread sticks (4″ long)
1 cup vegetable soup
Diet soft drink

Snack

2 cups popcorn (air-popped or microwaved)
8 oz. fruit juice

Dinner

Tossed salad, with 1 tablespoon oil and vinegar dressing
3 oz. flounder sauteed with 1 teaspoons margarine
1/2 cup cooked beets
1/2 cup steamed cauliflower
1 slice dry whole wheat toast
8 oz. skim milk

DAY SIX

Breakfast

4 oz. orange or other juice
3/4 cup ready-to-eat cereal
1/2 banana
1 cup 1% low-fat milk
1 slice whole wheat toast
1 teaspoon margarine
Coffee or tea (sugar-free)

Lunch

3 oz. Virginia ham sandwich, on rye bread, with lettuce, tomato, and 1 teaspoon mayonnaise
Piece of fruit
8 oz. skim milk

Snack

8 oz. low-fat yogurt

Dinner

Tossed salad, with 1 tablespoon low-fat French dressing
3 oz. broiled steak
1/2 cup sauteed mushrooms
Baked potato (approx. 2 1/2 × 4 3/4″)
1 teaspoon margarine
4 steamed asparagus spears
8 oz. skim milk

DAY SEVEN

Breakfast

Piece of fruit
1 scrambled egg
1 toasted bagel
2 teaspoons margarine
8 oz. skim milk
Coffee or tea (sugar-free)

Lunch

3 oz. turkey sandwich on whole wheat bread with lettuce, tomato and 1 teaspoon mayonnaise
Fruit
8 oz. skim milk

Snack

2 graham crackers
8 oz. skim milk

Dinner

Tossed salad, with 1 tablespoon oil and vinegar dressing
1 1/2 slices lean roast pork loin (approx. 3 oz.)
1/2 cup oven-browned potatoes
1/2 cup peas
1/2 cup sweetened applesauce
8 oz. skim milk
1/2 cup strawberries topped with 1/4 cup yogurt

SEVEN-DAY MEAL PLAN FOR . . .

. . . MOST ADULT FEMALES who wish to MAINTAIN their current weight (approximately 1600 calories daily)

DAY ONE

Breakfast

1/2 cup orange juice (or: piece of fruit)
3/4 cup ready-to-eat cereal
8 oz. 1% low-fat milk
Coffee or tea

Lunch

Peanut butter and jelly sandwich with 2 tablespoons peanut butter and 2 tablespoons jelly
Apple
3 carrot sticks
3 celery sticks
8 oz. 1% low fat milk

Snack

2 crackers
8 oz. 1% low fat milk

Dinner

3 oz. filet of haddock, pan-browned with 2 teaspoons margarine
Tossed salad, with 2 tablespoons low-cal dressing
1/2 cup steamed fresh broccoli with lemon
1/2 small baked potato with 1 teaspoon margarine
1/2 cup fruit salad
4 oz. 1% low fat milk, coffee, or tea

DAY TWO

Breakfast

1/2 cup fruit juice
1/2 banana
3/4 cup ready-to-eat cereal
8 oz. 1% low-fat milk
Coffee or tea

Lunch

2 oz. grilled cheese sandwich, on whole wheat bread, grilled with 1 teaspoon margarine or butter
Orange
4 oz. 1% low fat milk

Snack

2 cups popcorn (air-popped or microwaved)
8 oz. 1% low fat milk

Dinner

Tossed lettuce and tomato salad, with 2 tablespoons low-cal French dressing
2 slices roast beef (approx. 4 oz.)
1/2 cup mashed potatoes
1 teaspoon margarine
1/2 cup fresh zucchini, sauteed with onion
Dinner roll
8 oz. 1% low fat milk

DAY THREE

Breakfast

1/4 cantaloupe melon (or: other fruit)
1/2 cup cooked cereal (instant or quick)
8 oz. 1% low-fat milk
1 slice whole wheat toast
1 teaspoon margarine
Coffee or tea

Lunch

Tuna salad sandwich on roll (approx. 1/2 cup tuna, 1 teaspoon mayonnaise)
3 tomato wedges
Piece of fruit
8 oz. 1% low fat milk

Snack

1 oz. cheese
2 saltine crackers
8 oz. iced tea (sugar-free) or diet soft drink

Dinner

2 oz. broiled breast of chicken
Tossed salad, with 1 tablespoon oil and vinegar dressing
Baked potato (small)
1 teaspoon margarine
1/2 cup steamed broccoli with lemon and parsley
8 oz. 1% low fat milk

DAY FOUR

Breakfast

4 oz. orange juice (or: other fruit juice)
1/2 cup ready-to-eat cereal
1 cup 1% low-fat milk
1/2 cup fresh fruit
Coffee or tea

Lunch

2 oz. sliced chicken sandwich on whole wheat bread with lettuce, tomato, and 1 teaspoon mayonnaise
Piece of fruit
8 oz. 1% low fat milk

Snack

1/8 cup shelled almonds (approx. 20)
4 oz. 1% low fat milk

Dinner

Tossed salad, with 1 tablespoon oil and vinegar dressing
2 oz. broiled pork chop
1/2 cup cooked rice
1 teaspoon margarine
1/2 cup applesauce
1/2 cup cooked green beans
8 oz. 1% low-fat milk

DAY FIVE

Breakfast

4 oz. orange juice (or: other fruit juice)
2 slices French toast with diet syrup
8 oz. 1% low-fat milk
Coffee or tea

Lunch

1/2 cup cottage cheese with fruit on lettuce
2 bread sticks (4″ long)
1 cup vegetable soup
4 oz. 1% low fat milk

Snack

2 cups popcorn (air-popped or microwaved)
8 oz. juice

Dinner

Tossed salad, with 1 tablespoon oil and vinegar dressing
2 oz. flounder sauteed with 1 teaspoon margarine
1/2 cup cooked beets
1/2 cup steamed cauliflower
4 oz. 1% low fat milk

DAY SIX

Breakfast

4 oz. orange juice (or: other fruit juice)
1/2 cup ready-to-eat cereal
1/2 banana
1 cup 1% low-fat milk
Coffee or tea

Lunch

2 oz. Virginia ham sandwich, on rye bread with lettuce, tomato, and 1 teaspoon mayonnaise
Piece of fruit
8 oz. 1% low fat milk

Snack

1/2 cup low-fat yogurt

Dinner

Tossed salad, with 1 tablespoon low-fat French dressing
2 oz. broiled steak
1/2 cup sauteed mushrooms
Baked potato (2 1/2″ *x* 4 3/4″)
1 teaspoon margarine
4 steamed asparagus spears
8 oz. 1% low fat milk

DAY SEVEN

Breakfast

Piece of fruit
1 scrambled egg
1/2 toasted bagel
1 teaspoon margarine
8 oz. 1% low-fat milk
Coffee or tea

Lunch

2 oz. turkey sandwich, on whole wheat bread with lettuce, tomato and 1 teaspoon mayonnaise
Piece of fruit
8 oz. 1% low fat milk

Snack

2 graham crackers
8 oz. 1% low-fat milk

Dinner

Tossed salad, with 1 tablespoon oil and vinegar dressing
1 1/2 slices lean roast pork loin (approx. 3 oz.)
1/2 cup oven-browned potatoes
1/2 cup peas
1/2 cup regular applesauce
8 oz. 1% low fat milk
1/2 cup strawberries topped with 1/4 cup low-fat yogurt

SEVEN-DAY MEAL PLAN FOR . . .

. . . MOST ADULT FEMALES who wish to REDUCE their current weight (approximately 1200 calories daily)

DAY ONE

Breakfast

1/2 cup orange juice
3/4 cup ready-to-eat cereal
8 oz. skim milk
Coffee or tea (sugar-free)

Lunch

1/2 peanut butter and jelly sandwich with 1 tablespoon peanut butter and 1 tablespoon jelly
Apple
3 carrot sticks
3 celery sticks
Diet soft drink

Snack

1 cup low-fat yogurt

Dinner

3 oz. filet of haddock, pan-browned with 2 teaspoons margarine
Tossed salad with 2 tablespoons low-cal dressing
1/2 cup steamed fresh broccoli with lemon
1/2 small baked potato with 1 teaspoon margarine
1/2 cup fruit salad
Iced tea (sugar-free)
8 oz. skim milk

DAY TWO

Breakfast

1/2 cup grapefruit (or: other fruit juice)
1/2 cup ready-to-eat cereal
8 oz. skim milk
Coffee or tea (sugar-free)

Lunch

1/2 grilled cheese sandwich, with 1 oz. cheese, 1 slice whole wheat bread, grilled with 1 teaspoon margarine
Orange
8 oz. skim milk

Snack

2 cups popcorn (air-popped or microwaved)
Diet soft drink

Dinner

Tossed lettuce and tomato salad, with 2 tablespoons low-cal French dressing
1 1/2 slices roast beef (approx. 3 oz.)
1/2 cup mashed potatoes
1 teaspoon margarine
1 cup fresh zucchini, sauteed with onion
Dinner roll
8 oz. skim milk

DAY THREE

Breakfast

1/4 cantaloupe melon or other fruit
1/2 cup cooked cereal (instant or quick)
8 oz. skim milk
Coffee or tea (sugar-free)

Lunch

Tuna salad sandwich on roll (approx. 1/2 cup tuna, 2 teaspoons mayonnaise)
3 tomato wedges
Apple or other fruit
8 oz. skim milk

Snack

2 graham crackers
8 oz. skim milk

Dinner

3 oz. broiled breast of chicken
Tossed salad, with 1 tablespoon oil and vinegar dressing
Baked potato (small)
1 teaspoon margarine or butter
1/2 cup steamed broccoli with lemon and parsley
4 oz. skim milk

DAY FOUR

Breakfast

4 oz. orange juice (or: other fruit juice)
1/2 cup ready-to-eat cereal
8 oz. skim milk
Coffee or tea (sugar-free)

Lunch

2 oz. sliced chicken sandwich on whole wheat bread with lettuce, tomato, and 1 teaspoon mayonnaise
Piece of fruit
8 oz. 1% low-fat milk

Snack

10 shelled almonds
4 oz. skim milk

Dinner

Tossed salad, with 2 tablespoons low-cal dressing
2 oz. broiled pork chop
1/2 cup cooked rice
1 teaspoon margarine
1/2 cup applesauce
1/2 cup cooked fresh green beans
8 oz. skim milk

DAY FIVE

Breakfast

Piece of fruit
1 slice French toast, with diet syrup
8 oz. skim milk
Coffee or tea (sugar-free)

Lunch

1/2 cup cottage cheese with fruit on lettuce
2 bread sticks (4″ long)
1 cup vegetable soup
4 oz. skim milk

Snack

2 cups popcorn (air-popped or microwaved)
4 oz. fruit juice

Dinner

Tossed salad, with diet dressing
2 oz. flounder sauteed with 2 teaspoons margarine
1/2 cup cooked beets
1/2 cup steamed cauliflower
8 oz. skim milk

DAY SIX

Breakfast

4 oz. orange juice (or: other fruit juice)
1/2 cup ready-to-eat cereal
8 oz. skim milk
Coffee or tea (sugar-free)

Lunch

1/2 sandwich made with: 2 oz. Virginia ham, slice rye bread, lettuce and tomato, and 1 teaspoon mayonnaise
Piece of fruit
8 oz. skim milk

Snack

1/2 cup low-fat yogurt

Dinner

Tossed salad, with 1 tablespoon low-fat French dressing
3 oz. broiled steak
1/2 cup sauteed mushrooms (prepared in Teflon pan)
1/2 medium baked potato
1 teaspoon margarine
4 steamed asparagus spears
1/2 cup ice cream
Coffee or tea (sugar-free)

DAY SEVEN

Breakfast

4 oz. orange juice (or: other fruit juice)
1 scrambled egg
1/2 toasted bagel
1 teaspoon margarine
8 oz. skim milk
Coffee or tea (sugar-free)

Lunch

1/2 sandwich made with: 2 oz. turkey, 1 slice whole wheat bread, lettuce and tomato, 1 teaspoon mayonnaise
Piece of fruit
8 oz. skim milk

Snack

1 graham cracker
4 oz. skim milk

Dinner

Tossed salad, with 1 tablespoon low-fat French dressing
1 slice lean roast pork loin (approx. 2 oz.)
1/2 cup oven-browned potatoes
1/2 cup peas
1/2 cup unsweetened applesauce
8 oz. skim milk
1/2 cup strawberries

Notes

Chapter One

1. E.V. McCollum, *A History of Nutrition.* Houghton Mifflin Co. Boston, 1957.

2. M. Pyke, *Food and Society.* John Murray. London, 1968.

3. Alfred Harper, *Nutrition: From Myth and Magic to Science. Nutrition Today,* volume 23, number 1, February 1988.

Chapter Six

1. *Smoking and Health: Report of the Advisory Committee to the Surgeon General of the Public Health Service.* D.H.E.W. publication number (P.H.S.) 1103. US Government Printing Office, 1964. Also: *Smoking and Health: A Report of the Surgeon General.* D.H.E.W. publication number (P.H.S.) 79-50066. U.S. Government Printing Office, 1979.

Chapter Seven

1. Keys, A., Anderson, J.T., and Grande, F., *Serum Cholesterol Response to Changes in the Diet.* Metabolism 14: 747-787, 1965. Also: Kannel, W.B. and Gordon, T., *The Framingham Study. An Epidemiological Investigation of Cardiovascular Disease. Section 24: The Framingham Diet Study: Diet and the Regulation of Serum Cholesterol.* D.H.E.W. Report. U.S. Government Printing Office, 1970.

2. Nichols, A.B., Ravenscroft, C., Lamphiear, D.E., and Ostrander, L.D., *Daily Nutritional Intake and Serum Lipid Levels. The Tecumseh Study.* American Journal of Clinical Nutrition 29: 1384-1392, 1976.

3. Shekelle, R.B., Shyrock, A.M., Paul, O., Lepper, M., Stamler, J., Liu, S., and Raynor, W.J., *Diet, Serum Cholesterol, and Death From Coronary Heart Disease: The Western Electric Study.* New England Journal of Medicine 304: 65-70, 1981. Also: Hjermann, I., Velve Byre, K., Holme, I., and Leren, P., *Effect of Diet and Smoking Intervention on the Incidence of Coronary Heart Disease. Report from the Oslo Study Group of a Randomised Trial in Healthy Men.* Lancet ii: 1303-1310, 1981. Also: Frick, M.H., Elo, O., Happa, K., et al., *Helsinki Heart Study: Primary-Prevention Trial with Gemfibrozil in Middle-Aged men with Dyslipidemia.* New England Journal of Medicine 317:1237-1245, 1987. Also: Olson, R.E., *Mass Intervention vs Screening and Selective Intervention for Prevention of CHD.* Journal of the American Medical Association 255: 2204-2207, 1986.

4. Taylor, William, et al., *Cholesterol Reduction and Life Expectancy: A Model Incorporating Multiple Risk Factors.* Annals of Internal Medicine, 106: 605, 1987.

Chapter Eight

1. *Indications for Cholesterol Testing in Children,* Pediatrics, January 81:141, 1989

2. Oliver, M.F., *Serum Cholesterol—the Knave of Hearts and the Joker,* Lancet, ii, 1090-1095, 1981.

Chapter Nine

1. Stare, Fredrick, and Whelan, Elizabeth, *The Harvard Square Diet.* Prometheus Books, 1987.

Appendix:

Specific Nutrients and Their Functions

Glossary

Recommended Reading

Specific Nutrients and Their Functions

CALCIUM

Where can you find it?

Milk, cheese, ice cream, cottage cheese (less calcium than regular cheese), broccoli, oysters, shrimp, salmon, clams, cabbage.

Greens: turnip, collards, Kale, mustard.

(Also: "hard" water.)

What does it do?

Needed for structure of bones and teeth. Needed for healthy nerves and muscle activity.

Essential in blood clotting.

Needed in healing wounds and broken bones.

CARBOHYDRATES

Where can you find them?

Flours, cereals, breads, cakes crackers, rice, noodles, macaroni, spaghetti, sugars, syrups, jellies, honey.

Some fruits and vegetables such as dried fruits, sweetened fruits, dried legumes, potatoes, corn, lima beans, and bananas.

Cellulose and fibers.

What do they do?

Primary source of energy for the body.

Primary energy source for the brain and nervous tissue.

Protects protein—spares the body from using protein to meet energy needs.

Complex carbohydrate is needed for bulk and proper elimination, and the normal growth of bacteria in the lower intestine.

COPPER

Where can you find it?

Meats (particularly liver), shellfish.

Nuts, raisins, dried legumes, cereal, cocoa, chocolate.

What does it do?

Active in synthesis of hemoglobin and metabolism of iron.

Active in maintenance of normal blood vessels.

FATS

Where can you find them?

Fat from beef, lamb, and pork; butter, margarine, lard, salad oil, hydrogenated shortening; cream, milk, cheese (except those made with skim milk); fried foods, pastries, chocolates, and rich desserts.

What do they do?

Provide concentrated form of energy for the body.

Carry the fat-soluble vitamins A, D, and E into the body; provide protection for the various vital organs and insulation for the body; increase palatability of food; provide "satisfaction"—delay onset of hunger.

FLUORIDE

Where can you find it?

Fluoridated water.

Many teas.

What does it do?

Promotes good dental health.

Aids in prevention of osteoporosis.

IODIDE

Where can you find it?

Iodized salt (the best source).

Seafoods and foods grown along the seacoast.

What does it do?

Needed to make the hormone thyroxine, which regulates the use of energy in the body.

Prevents goiter.

IRON

Where can you find it?

Liver, lean meats, poultry, shellfish, egg yolk, clams, oysters.

Green leafy vegetables, whole-grain and enriched cereals and breads, legumes and nuts, molasses.

Certain fruits such as peaches, apricots, prunes, grapes, raisins.

What does it do?

Needed to form hemoglobin, which carries oxygen from the lungs to the body cells.

A component of many enzymes.

MAGNESIUM

Where can you find it?

Whole-grain cereals, potatoes, nuts, legumes, meats.

(Also: "hard" water.)

(Dietary deficiency unlikely.)

What does it do?

Needed for structure of bones and teeth.

Helps transmit nerve impulses.

Helps muscle contraction.

Activates enzymes needed for carbohydrate and energy metabolism.

PHOSPHORUS

Where can you find it?

Meats, milk, cheese, ice cream, meat, poultry, fish, whole-grain cereals, nuts, legumes.

(Dietary deficiency unlikely if diet contains enough protein and calcium.)

What does it do?

Needed in combination with calcium for bones and teeth.

Needed for enzymes used in energy metabolism.

Regulates the balance between acids and bases in the body.

POTASSIUM

Where can you find it?

Citrus fruits, cantaloupe, bananas, apricots, other fresh fruits, fruit juices, vegetables, meat, fish, and cereals.

What does it do?

Aids in synthesis of protein.

Helps maintain fluid balance.

Required for healthy nerves and muscles.

Needed for enzyme reactions.

PROTEIN

Where can you find it?

Meat, fish, poultry, egg white, milk, cheese.

Dried beans and peas, peanut butter, nuts, bread and cereal have nutritionally incomplete proteins but are adequate if served with milk, eggs, or meat.

What does it do?

Constituent of all body cells.

Needed for: structure of red blood cells (hemoglobin); antibodies to fight infection and disease; and enzymes and hormones to regulate body processes.

Needed for growth, maintenance and repair of tissue. Regulates amount of water present in the spaces between body cells.

SODIUM (SALT)

Where can you find it?

Table salt.

Meat, fish, poultry, milk, eggs.

Foods where salt is a preservative (ham, bacon, olives, fish, etc.).

What does it do?

Helps maintain fluid balance.

Keeps balance of acids and bases in body.

Helps in the absorption of other nutrients.

VITAMIN A

Where can you find it?

Liver, kidney (excellent sources), egg yolk, dark-green leafy and deep-yellow vegetables, tomatoes, butter, fortified margarine, whole milk and cheese made from whole milk and fortified skim milk.

What does it do?

Needed for growth, healthy skin, bones, and teeth, particularly for children.

Helps maintain good vision, especially in poor light.

Helps body resist infection.

VITAMIN B GROUP: BIOTIN

Where can you find it?

Meats, egg yolk, legumes, nuts.

What does it do?

Interrelated with functions of other nutrients in the vitamin B group.

VITAMIN B GROUP: CYANOCOBALAMIN (Vitamin B_{12})

Where can you find it?

Provided only by foods of animal origin: meats (especially liver and kidney), fish, milk, eggs, cheese.

Does not occur in fruits, vegetables, or cereals. Vegetarians beware!

What does it do?

Needed for production of red blood cells in bone marrow.

Needed for building new proteins in the body.

Needed for normal functioning of nervous tissue.

VITAMIN B GROUP: FOLACIN OR FOLIC ACID

Where can you find it?

Variety of foods of animal and vegetable origin, particularly glandular meats, such as liver, but also in green leafy vegetables, many fruits, eggs, and whole-grain cereals.

What does it do?

Necessary for the development of red blood cells.

Needed for normal metabolism of carbohydrates, proteins, and fats.

VITAMIN B GROUP: NIACIN

Where can you find it?

Poultry, meats, fish, and organ meats.

Peanuts, peanut butter, legumes, dark green leafy vegetables, potatoes, whole-grain or enriched breads, cereals.

What does it do?

Needed for healthy nervous system, healthy skin, normal digestion.

Helps cells use oxygen to release energy.

Needed to use protein in the body.

Needed for normal growth.

VITAMIN B GROUP: PANTOTHENIC ACID

Where can you find it?

Meats, liver, kidney, heart, fish, eggs, vegetables, legumes, whole grains.

What does it do?

Active in breakdown of carbohydrates, fats and proteins for the production of energy.

Active in synthesis of amino acids, fatty acids, sterols, and steroid hormones.

VITAMIN B GROUP: PYRIDOXINE (Vitamin B_6)

Where can you find it?

Meats (especially pork and the glandular meats), lamb veal, liver, kidney, wheat germ, whole-grain cereals, soybeans, peanuts, corn.

What does it do?

Prevents certain forms of anemia

Needed for normal utilization of copper and iron.

VITAMIN B GROUP: RIBOFLAVIN (Vitamin B_2)

Where can you find it?

Milk and cheese are the best sources.

Liver, kidney and heart, other meats, eggs, green leafy vegetables, enriched breads and cereals.

What does it do?

Constituent of many enzymes needed to use protein, fats and carbohydrates for energy and building tissues.

Maintains healthy skin, especially around the mouth, nose and eyes.

VITAMIN B GROUP: THIAMINE (Vitamin B_1)

Where can you find it?

Whole-grain products or enriched breads and cereals.

Meats (especially pork), poultry, fish.

Liver, dry beans and peas, soybeans, peanuts, egg yolk.

What does it do?

Helps to use carbohydrates for energy in the body.

Helps maintain healthy nervous system.

VITAMIN C (ASCORBIC ACID)

Where can you find it?

Citrus fruits, strawberries, tomatoes, cantaloupe, broccoli, raw green vegetables, cabbage, boiled potato, canned or frozen citrus fruit juices.

What does it do?

Needed for building the material that holds cells together.

Needed for health of teeth, gums and blood vessels.

Helps body resist infection and aids in healing wounds (but is not effective in the prevention or treatment of the common cold).

Helps synthesize hormones to regulate body functions.

Improves iron absorption.

VITAMIN D

Where can you find it?

Fortified milk, egg yolk, liver, fish (herring, sardines, tuna, salmon).

With direct sunlight on the skin the body can manufacture its own.

What does it do?

Needed for the absorption and utilization of calcium and phosphorus.

Needed for healthy bones and sound teeth.

VITAMIN E

Where can you find it?

Green leafy vegetables, nuts, legumes, salad oils, shortenings, margarines, meat, fish, milk, eggs and many other sources.

What does it do?

Helps protect vitamin A and polyunsaturated fatty acids.

Protects red blood cells.

(Has nothing to do with sex or heart disease!)

VITAMIN K

Where can you find it?

Synthesized naturally by bacteria in the human intestinal tract.

Minimal amounts in green leaves of spinach, kale and cabbage; cauliflower, pork liver.

What does it do?

Promotes normal blood clotting.

WATER

Where can you find it?

Innumerable direct and indirect sources.

What does it do?

Water acts in many ways to keep us healthy. It is a practical medium for transporting nutrients to the various cells of the body and for removing the cellular waste products. In addition, water serves as a cushioning device since it is not readily compressible and acts additionally as a lubricant in body movement. Water is also an essential compound in the chemical reactions of digestion, breaking down carbohydrates, splitting glycerol from fatty acids, among other processes.

Water gives structure to the body, retaining the shape of cells. Some 40 percent of body weight is water located within cells. Finally, water serves as a temperature-regulating substance: the evaporation of water from the lungs and skin removes heat from the body. If you want to demonstrate your water loss from your lungs, breathe into a glass. There you will have your evidence.

ZINC

Where can you find it?

Green leafy foods, fruit, whole grains, meats, and vegetables.

What does it do?

Helps in wound healing. Component of many enzymes.

Essential for normal growth and development.

GLOSSARY

Adipose: A medical term meaning fatty. Usually used in reference to the animal tissue that stores fat—as, adipose tissue.

Amino Acids: The basic chemical compounds that when properly combined make up proteins—the building blocks of proteins. They are organic compounds containing nitrogen as well as carbon, hydrogen, and oxygen. There are some twenty-two amino acids, eight of which are called "essential" because the body cells cannot make them and hence it is essential that they be received from the foods of the diet. The other amino acids are also obtained from foods, but the body can also make them, principally in the liver, from other dietary ingredients.

Anemia: A blood disorder in which there is either an insufficient number of red blood cells or a reduced amount of hemoglobin, the oxygen-carrying pigment of the red blood cells, or both.

Arteriosclerosis: A thickening and occasionally a hardening, due to calcification, of the walls of arteries and capillaries resulting in a loss of elasticity of the vessel wall and a narrowing of the size of the vessel.

Ascorbic Acid: Another name for vitamin C, the vitamin historically associated with the disease called scurvy. Ascorbic acid is particularly necessary for healthy gums, as well as many other body tissues, because of its role in the formation of connective tissue. Fresh fruits (especially citrus) and vegetables are the principal sources of this vitamin.

Atherosclerosis: A type of arteriosclerosis characterized by fatty deposits containing cholesterol in the inner lining of arteries. It is the type of arteriosclerosis usually present when one has coronary heart disease, a stroke, or an aneurysm.

Balanced Diet: A diet made up of a variety of foods from the different food groups (Basic Four) so that all the many nutrients are obtained in proper or balanced amounts.

Basic Four: A term used to describe a classification of foods into four groups that supply certain categories of nutrients:

Fruits and vegetables
Cereals and foods made from them, and potatoes
Milk and related products
Meat and meat alternatives

By eating certain quantities of foods from each group one is likely to receive a "balanced diet"—that is, a diet providing all nutrients in proper amounts.

Bran: The coarse outer coat of grains. In the diet it provides bulk, and this is important to prevent constipation.

Calcium: A mineral nutrient, essential for bone and teeth formation, and a variety of metabolic processes such as the clotting of blood, beating of the heart, and other types of muscular contraction, and the conduction of impulses along nerve fibers.

Calorie: The unit by which the energy value of food is measured. The calorie, or energy value of foods, is defined as the amount of heat energy required to raise 1000 grams (approximately one quart) of water one degree Centigrade. In practice, the calorie value is determined by calculation using the composition of the food in terms of fat, protein, and carbohydrate. Each gram of fat produces nine calories, and each gram of protein and carbohydrate, four calories.

Carbohydrate: A group of organic chemical substances containing carbon, hydrogen, and oxygen that are found in foods and utilized by the body for energy. Starch and sugars are the common carbohydrates. Cereals and root vegetables are the common food sources of starches.

Caries: Tooth decay.

Carotene: Yellow compounds of carbon and hydrogen found in yellow and green plants. Some carotenes are converted by the body into vitamin A. In green plants the yellow color is masked by a larger concentration of the green pigment known as chlorophyll.

Cell: The structural and functional microscopic unit of plant and animal organisms.

Cellulose: A complex carbohydrate found in the fibrous parts of plants. It is poorly digested by humans and hence provides no calories. Cows, sheep, goats, and horses can digest cellulose and get energy from it.

Chemical: A chemical is any substance made up of elements. For example, two atoms of hydrogen and one of oxygen make a molecule of water (H_2O)—a chemical. One atom of sodium and one of chlorine make a molecule of table salt (NaCl)—a chemical. A number of atoms of hydrogen, oxygen, and carbon when combined in the proper way make a molecule of cholesterol, and thousands of other chemicals.

Cholesterol: The commonest member of a group of compounds called "sterols." These are composed of carbon, hydrogen, and oxygen. Cholesterol is present in all animal tissues but not in plant tissues, though the latter contain similar sterols. Cholesterol is present in many foods, but only foods of animal origin. Egg yolk, sweetbreads, liver, and brains are especially rich sources. It is also made by the body. It is an essential raw material for the manufacture by the body of sex and adrenal hormones, of vitamin D, and is a constituent of the abnormal deposits in the inner layer of arteries giving rise to atherosclerosis.

Colitis: Inflammation of the colon, which is the wider part of the intestine making up the latter half of this organ.

Coronary: Referring to the arteries within the heart and which supply the heart muscle tissue with nourishment and oxygen.

Deficiency Disease: A disease resulting from the inadequate intake (a deficiency) of an essential nutrient. Thus scurvy is due to a deficiency of ascorbic acid, pellagra to a deficiency of niacin, and kwashiorkor to a deficiency of protein.

Desirable Weight: That weight at which most people will live longest. Insurance actuarial data indicate that average weight at age twenty-five years for each sex and for any given height is best for longevity, and the Metropolitan Life Insurance Company termed this "desirable weight." Prior to 1945 this weight was called "ideal weight."

Digestion: The breaking down of foods into simple components in the digestive tract and their absorption into the blood. Proteins are digested to peptides and amino acids, fats to fatty acids and glycerol, and carbohydrates to dextrins and sugars.

Edema: An accumulation of abnormal amounts of fluid in the inter-tissue spaces of the body, between cells, which results in a swelling.

Edible: A term applied to that portion of food that is fit (or ready) to eat.

Emulsification: The process of breaking large fat particles into smaller ones that will remain suspended as small particles in another liquid—as, for example, the small particles of fat suspended in homogenized milk.

Endogenous: A term used to refer to substances originating from within or inside the cells or tissues as contrasted with substances reaching tissues from outside the body. Thus endogenous cholesterol refers to the cholesterol manufactured by the body out of other compounds, and exogenous cholesterol refers to cholesterol obtained from foods.

Energy: In nutrition the caloric equivalent of the heat and work necessary to maintain the temperature of the body and permit muscular contraction and thus perform work.

Enrich: To add one or more nutrients to a food to bring its content of those nutrients up to the approximate level in the food before processing.

Enzyme: A substance, protein in nature, formed in living cells, which brings about and greatly accelerates chemical changes but does not enter into the change. Many enzymes consist of specific vitamins combined with specific proteins.

Essential: A term used to refer to specific nutrients required for some body reactions necessary for life and which must be supplied from foods because the body cannot make these nutrients from other dietary substances. Thus, lysine is an "essential" amino acid essential for growth, and must be received in adequate amounts from the diet; however, glycine, another amino acid, is not essential in the diet, as the body can make it from other components of the diet. Copper and iron are mineral nutrients essential for the formation of hemoglobin, the red coloring matter of the blood that is needed to carry oxygen to the cells of the body, obviously an essential function. Fluoride is a mineral nutrient essential for the formation of dental enamel that has a chemical and physical structure that provides maximum resistance to decay.

Exogenous: A term used to refer to substances originating outside the cells or tissues of the body. For example: exogenous cholesterol refers to dietary sources of cholesterol, not that made within the body, which is called endogenous.

Fat: A chemical compound composed of three fatty acids combined with a molecule of glycerol. Fats are either animal or vegetable in origin and may be solid or liquid. They also may be man-made—that is, synthesized in the laboratory.

Fat Soluble: Refers to substances that do not dissolve in water but do in fats, oils, or in fat solvents. For example, vitamins A and D are fat-soluble. In nature they are found dissolved in butter fat, as contrasted with vitamin C, which is water-soluble and found dissolved in the watery juice of citrus fruit.

Fatty Acids: Organic acids that combine with glycerol to form fat. They are usually classified as "saturated" or "unsaturated." Fatty acids are chains of carbon atoms to which are attached two hydrogen atoms for each carbon atom, and at the end of the chain are two oxygen atoms, one combined with carbon and the other with carbon and hydrogen. If all the hydrogens that can be attached to the carbon atoms are present in the chain, the acid is called saturated. If two adjacent carbons are each lacking a hydrogen, a "double bond" results and the acid is considered unsaturated—that is, hydrogen can be added at the site of the double bond. If there is one double bond in the chain the fatty acid is called monounsaturated. Olive oil is an example of an oil containing a good deal of monounsaturated fatty acid, the specific acid being oleic acid. If there are two or more double bonds the substance is called polyunsaturated. The most common polyunsaturated fatty acid (P.U.F.A.) is called linoliec acid. It is found in corn, cottonseed, safflower, soy oil, where it makes up about half or more of the total fatty acids. Linoleic acid is an "essential" fatty acid since it must be furnished by the food we eat. Linolenic and arachidonic are two other polyunsaturated fatty acids that are "essential."

Fluoridation: The adjustment of the mineral nutrient fluoride in a water supply, usually so that the concentration of fluoride will be one part of fluoride per million parts of water. Fluoridation is a public-health procedure that will dramatically reduce the amount of dental decay in children (and future adults).

Folic Acid: A vitamin of the B-complex group, and important in metabolism of the red blood cells and in certain enzyme reactions.

Food Additives: Chemical compounds added to foods to improve flavor, appearance, preservation, or nutritive qualities and thus provide better nutrition and economy through longer keeping qualities of the food.

Food Faddist: One who attaches unusual health-promoting properties to a specific food or diet, usually for a specific disease or group of diseases, and in the absence of any generally accepted scientific evidence.

Food Quack: One who pretends to know something about foods and nutrition, generally in relation to human health, but who has had little or no training in these subjects and who is not recognized or respected by those who have studied and contributed to this area of science.

Fortify: To add one or more nutrients to a food so that it contains more of the nutrient than the food provides as it occurs in nature. For example, milk is often fortified with vitamin D, and margarine with vitamin A.

Galactose: A simple sugar derived from milk sugar or lactose, it constitutes half of the molecule of lactose.

Glucose: A simple sugar that makes up half of the molecule of sucrose (ordinary table sugar). It is also the type of sugar present in the blood and which is utilized (metabolized) by the body to yield energy.

Gram: A unit of weight in the metric system. One gram is approximately 1/28 of an ounce.

Iodide: A mineral nutrient essential for the proper functioning of the thyroid gland as it is a part of the molecule of the hormone thyroxin, made by this endocrine gland.

Iron: A mineral nutrient, necessary for the formation of hemoglobin, the substance in red blood cells necessary for carrying oxygen to the cells of the body.

Kwashiorkor: The name of a disease occurring in children generally between one and five years of age in many of the underdeveloped areas of the world. It is due to lack of adequate quantities of good quality protein, is frequently a fatal disease, and is one of the leading causes of death in this age group in underdeveloped countries.

Linoleic Acid: See fatty acids.

Linolenic Acid: See fatty acids.

Lipid: Fat or fatlike substances.

Metabolism: A term used to describe all chemical changes that occur in living matter.

Milligram: A measure of weight in the metric system, 1/1000th of a gram.

Minerals: Naturally occurring inorganic elements, some of which are essential to life in animals and plants. The minerals commonly given consideration in human nutrition are sodium, potassium, calcium, phosphorus, iron, iodide, copper, magnesium, cobalt, chloride, manganese, fluoride, sulfur, selenium, zinc, and molybdenum.

Niacin: A member of the B-complex vitamins. Historically, it is associated with the prevention of pellagra.

Nutrient: A chemical compound needed for specific functions in the nourishment of the body. Protein, amino acids, fat, sugar, starch, minerals, vitamins, water are all nutrients. There are some fifty known nutrients.

Obesity: Excessive body weight due to the presence of a surplus of body fat, sometimes defined as 20 percent or more above "desirable" weight.

Oils: Any fat that remains liquid at room temperature. Most of the common edible oils are of vegetable origin and contain a fair amount of saturated, monounsaturated, or polyunsaturated fatty acids.

Overweight: Sometimes defined as 10 to 20 percent over "desirable" weight, as contrasted with obese, which is 20 percent or more above "desirable" weight.

Phenylketonuria: A hereditary disease in which there is a lack of the specific enzyme needed to use (metabolize) the amino acid phenylalanine. This disease results in an increased amount of phenylpyruvic acid in the blood and urine and may damage parts of the brain, causing mental retardation. The disease is usually diagnosed in infancy or early childhood.

Riboflavin: A water-soluble vitamin of the B-complex (B_2) that is important in many enzyme reactions, particularly those involving the transfer of energy from food to the cells.

Roughage: The indigestible material found in food. In vegetables, it is called cellulose, bran, or fiber; in animals, it is connective tissue.

Saccharin: A white crystalline compound of high degree of sweetness used as a substitute for sugar. It has no caloric value.

Sodium: A mineral nutrient involved in many of the fluid systems of the body. The most common food source is table salt.

Sterol: Fatlike or fat-soluble compounds with a somewhat complex structure. Cholesterol and vitamin D are common examples of the sterols.

Synthetic: Refers to the process of making or "building up" a compound by the union of simpler compounds or their elements. Common usage assigns this term to compounds made in the laboratory, or in industry, as opposed to compounds made by the body.

Thiamin: One of the B-complex vitamins also known as vitamin B_1. Historically, it is associated with the prevention of the disease known as beriberi, which is common among those who eat large amounts of polished rice.

Tooth Enamel: The hard outer covering of the tooth made of inorganic material, mostly complex compounds of calcium and phosphates, and which is made more resistant to decay when fluoride is combined with the calcium and phosphates.

Vascular: Pertaining to, or full of, blood vessels.

Vitamin: One of a group of organic substances that in relatively small amounts are essential for life and growth. They are commonly divided into two groups on the basis of their solubility: the fat-soluble vitamins (A, D, E, and K); and the water-soluble vitamins (ascorbic acid or vitamin C and the B-complex vitamins).

Vitamin A: A member of the fat-soluble vitamins. It is necessary for growth, vision, and healthy skin.

Vitamin B Complex: See individual B-vitamins—thiamin, riboflavin, niacin, and folic acid.

Vitamin C: See ascorbic acid.
Vitamin D: A fat-soluble vitamin—the "sunshine vitamin," important for building strong bones and teeth in that it favors the absorption of calcium. We usually get all we need by the action of sunlight in changing certain sterols in the skin into vitamin D. This is then transported by the blood to the liver, where it is stored for future use.
Vitamin E: A fat-soluble vitamin that helps protect Vitamin A and polyunsaturated fatty acids, and protects red blood cells.
Vitamin K: A fat-soluble vitamin needed for the clotting of blood. There are no good food sources of vitamin K. Most of it is obtained by absorbing it from bacteria that normally live and multiply in the large intestine.

Adapted, with permission, from EAT OK, FEEL OK!, published by Christopher Publishing.

Recommended Reading

Introductory Nutrition, Helen A. Guthrie, 7th Ed., Times Mirror/Mosby College Publishers, 1989.
Diet and Health: Implications for Reducing Chronic Disease Risk, Committee on Diet and Health, National Research Council, Washington, DC 20418, 1989; Executive Summary of 19 pages, Full Report of 996 pages.
The Surgeon General's Report on Nutrition and Health, U.S. Department of Health and Human Services, Public Health Service, 1988.
Promoting Health/Preventing Disease, U.S. Department of Health and Human Services, Public Health Service, 1988.
Annual Review of Nutrition, R.E. Olson, Editor, Annual Reviews, Inc., Palo Alto, CA, 1988.
The Paleolithic Prescription: A Program of Diet and Exercise and a Design for Living, S. Eaton, M. Shostak, and M. Konner, Harper and Row, 1988.
The California Nutrition Book, P. Saltman, J. Gurin, and I. Mothner, Little Brown and Co., Boston, 1987.
Fish and Human Health, W. E. M. Lands, Academic Press, Harcourt, Brace, Jovanovich, 1986.
Rx: Executive Diet—Sensible Nutrition for Today's Health-conscious Executives, F. J. Stare and V. Aronson, Christopher Publishing House, Norwell, MA, 1986.
Toxic Terror, E. Whelan, Jameson Books, Ottawa, IL, 1985.
Alcohol and the Fetus, H.L. Rosett and L. Weiner, Oxford University Press, 1984.
Present Knowledge in Nutrition, R.E. Olson, Editor, The Nutrition Foundation, Washington, DC, 1984.
Eat Better, Live Better, Reader's Digest Assoc., Inc., Pleasantville, New York, 1982.
Nutrition: A Manual for Medical Students and Physicians, 4th Ed., F.J. Stare, et al., the Upjohn Co., Kalamazoo, MI, 1980.

Index